COCAINE

From Dependency to Recovery

Cardwell C. Nuckols

 Human Services Institute, Inc.
Bradenton, Florida

Library of Congress Cataloging-in-Publication Data

    Nuckols, Cardwell C.
      Cocaine: from dependency to recovery.

      Bibliography: p.
      Includes index.
      1. Cocaine habit.   2. Cocaine habit--Treatment.
  I.   Title.
    RC568.C6N83 1987   616.86'4   87-61534
    ISBN 0-943519-00-4

Copyright 1987 by Cardwell C. Nuckols

Human Services Institute, Inc.
P.O. Box 14610
Bradenton, FL 34280

Development Editor: Lee Marvin Joiner, Ph.D.
Design and Production: Margaret E. Dickson
Cover Art and Design: Frank Cochrane Assoc.

Printed in the United States of America

Printing: 1 2 3 4 5 6 7 8 9   Year: 7 8 9 0 1 2

CONTENTS

FOREWORD

When a drug hits the market, there suddenly appears a rash of prophets, prognosticators, and pundits. Coupled with this fact are three traits of the American character:

We want things now;
We like simple answers; and
As a people who are basically pragmatic, if it works, use it;
if it doesn't, get rid of it.

Translated into language used in the field of sensory experience: if it gives pleasure, it is good; if it gives pain, it is bad.

Over the last few years, cocaine has assumed an ever increasing place in the center of the chemical dependency field, as well as in American culture. There has been a virtual outpouring of articles, books, and films either extolling its virtues or warning of its devastating and destructive nature.

In the campaign of 1986, Congress found "religion" in talking about drugs—particularly about cocaine and/or crack. I think it would be fair to say that there was a *media hype* which almost bordered on hysteria. Carwell Nuckols has written a book which, in my opinion, brings a well needed measure of sanity and a rational perspective to this issue. It does not purport to be the definitive answer, for at this time in our history, there is no definitive answer or conclusion to the cocaine story. Combining a mixture of his own experience, and the shared experiences of countless others, all seasoned with a solid knowledge of the issue (theoretical and applied), this book offers to both lay people and professionals, a challenge, a learning opportunity, and a true sense of hope. If read carefully, the individual will get a much clearer understanding of this oftentimes deadly universal problem. In truth, no one can say that it is NOT my problem, for everyone in this country is at risk from any individual who uses drugs, cocaine being just one of the many available to our citizenry today.

Mr. Nuckols is to be thanked for bringing such a clear, coherent exposition of this insidious and frightening issue to the attention of the people of this country.

As a doctor who has been working in the alcohol/drug abuse field for almost twenty-five years, I strongly recommend this book and thank Cardwell deeply for the privilege and the pleasure of having been allowed to write this brief foreword.

Jokichi Takamine, M.D.
Immediate Past Chairman,
AMA Task Force on Alcoholism

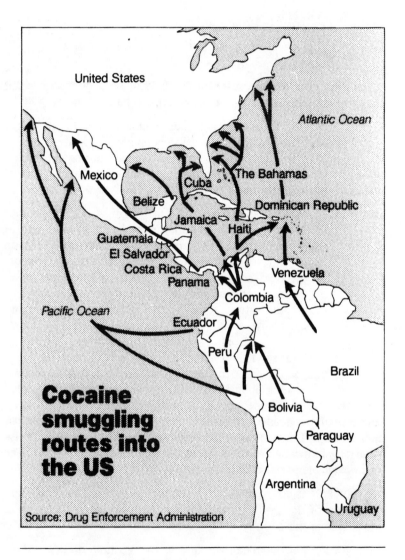

Cocaine smuggling routes into the US

United States

Atlantic Ocean

Mexico

Belize

Cuba

The Bahamas

Jamaica

Dominican Republic

Guatemala

Haiti

El Salvador

Costa Rica

Panama

Venezuela

Pacific Ocean

Colombia

Ecuador

Peru

Brazil

Bolivia

Paraguay

Argentina

Uruguay

Source: Drug Enforcement Administration

Remillard in The Christian Science Monitor ℗ 1987 TCSPS

PREFACE

COCAINE: From Dependency to Recovery is a book for anyone concerned with cocaine dependence. Therapists, counselors, physicians, nurses, concerned family members and people who think they have developed a cocaine dependency problem can find useful information here. The material in the book arises from my own research and experience, first as a cocaine dependent and later as a therapist engaged in the treatment of cocaine addiction. I have tried to provide the information and insights that I think will help other therapists, cocaine addicts and their families, and concerned laymen confront this serious human problem.

Some of the material in the book describes how therapists work with cocaine dependency. However, I must remind readers that experience, training, and supervision are crucial requisites for success as a therapist. No single book can provide all the answers, much less the experience. There is often a mystique surrounding the therapy process and a tendency to consider techniques "secret." However, therapy is an interaction between therapist and patient, directed in this instance toward the goal of recovering from an addiction. The more both participants in the process know about each other—their motives, assumptions, and objectives—the better the chance of recovery. Families of cocaine addicts should know everything they can about the treatment process in order to support rather than obstruct it. There aren't any secrets.

An aura of glamour and mystery surrounds cocaine. The mystique is heightened by special terms and concepts that create social distance between cocaine users and those uninvolved in "the cocaine culture." First, we should be aware that cocaine wasn't always considered "evil." There are classic stories conveying a positive image of cocaine use. For example, the man who designed the Statue of Liberty wrote a letter to a gentleman who produced a wine preparation laced with cocaine:

My dear Mr. Mariani:

If I had only had your magic elixir when I was designing the Statue of Liberty, the statue would have been at least 100 meters taller.

Consider Sigmund Freud and the glamour ascribed to his use of cocaine in psychiatric treatment. Freud treated many ailments with cocaine: dyspepsia, alcoholism, narcotics addiction, and depression. He even sent it to his lover to relieve her depression.

Robert Lewis Stevensen was treated with cocaine for tuberculosis. During his treatment he wrote *Dr. Jekyl and Mr. Hyde.* It is said that he wrote it in three days. Ironically, cocaine has become the Dr. Jekyl and Mr. Hyde of all drugs. No other substance I know of has the propensity to cause the problems this drug can.

There is much material available to readers on the bare facts about cocaine and the horror stories surrounding its use. It is relatively easy to learn about the pharmacology of the drug. Nevertheless, as some addicts cling to the power legends of cocaine, many "outsiders" including professional therapists and counselors, remain intimidated by the language and culture of cocaine addiction. For instance, anyone "have a summer cold?" Ever "eaten a doughnut in the bathroom" and gotten the white powder on your nose? Semantic barriers like these must be overcome if you want to understand and help the cocaine addict, as family member, friend, or therapist.

What is the cocaine addict like? People who have never been dependent on cocaine have no clear idea of its effects. If you are an alcohol counselor and recovering yourself, or if you have had trouble with marijuana, valium, or librium, you can relate to the experiences of people with similar drug dependency problems. If you are an alcoholic or have been drunk and hung over, you can sit down and know how a client feels. You can get right into their system and experience. But when a cocaine addict says, "I went out and copped an eight-ball last night," or "I went out basing and balling," you may say, "What was this person doing?" What is the cocaine addict's reality? Many people who would like to help, often therapists and counselors, are intimidated by the language of cocaine.

Without the language and shared experiences, you may look at the cocaine user in an entirely different light. He or she may offend and repel you. You can't penetrate their reality. Beyond this, the addict may begin to convey a sense of uniqueness or specialness. Attitudes, words and actions are chosen to say, "I am special."

Cocaine addicts want to be special. They seek power and control. When you try to establish communication and rapport there will be a test. If you don't know an "eight-ball" is an eighth of an ounce of cocaine (or 3.5 grams), if you don't know what "freebasing" is, don't know how to "fire up" cocaine, and don't understand colloquialisms such as "speed-balling" (cocaine laced with heroin) you will have difficulties.

Cocaine addicts don't perceive themselves as addicts. They see themselves as productive people. They don't like inpatient remedies. They like outpatient solutions. And they often want to talk about physical problems. It doesn't make any difference what type of person you're dealing with. It doesn't make any difference if they freebase cocaine or use it intravenously. The difference is in how we deal with them. Much of the content of *COCAINE* describes methods I have used to help cocaine addicts recover. In this book I try to portray a realistic picture of cocaine: the experience, the drug, addiction, and the hard realities of recovery.

One thing I stress is that counselors bear fifty percent of the responsibility for creating the motivation for the cocaine addict's recovery. I often hear counselors say, "Gee, I guess this person just needed a little more field research; they needed to go and fall on their face once or twice more." As a former director of several chemical dependency programs, it breaks my heart to hear this. When cocaine addicts insist on outpatient remedies, want to focus discussion on physical problems, and are unwilling to work hard with you to enter an inpatient environment, I think it is time to start planting some seeds. Help create the motivation for recovery.

I think of the case of a man who was attended a community seminar in Miami. He was in the back row and would get up and walk out every fifteen minutes. I assumed he was going to the bathroom, "eating some doughnuts," or something. I talked to him later and it was interesting. People who use cocaine put on a face, but they are basically lonely and desperate, with many problems. This man came up to me and said, "C.C., I like what you said. You talked about me today. I can see myself in all of what you've talked about. I've had a seizure, sinus problems, and upper respiratory tract infections for over four years now. I smuggle cocaine...just brought ten pounds of Freebase in from the Bahamas." This man continued, "Look, I don't want to talk about going into treatment, I don't want to talk about problems. All I want to know is what will happen to me next physically? And I want someone to talk to because, you see, its lonely here."

An agony was inside this man, but cocaine's grandiosity and the strange things it did to his mind were all there too. I talked to him for a little while. He came from an upper middle class family, a lawyer's son, and had been through college. He had a career and was in the process of "blowing" it all. He reminded me of another person I worked with who was a vice-president of a corporation. The first time I met him his family came to me for an intervention. He lived in a luxurious home. In nine months, he was selling cocaine on the street, living in the worst part of Chicago. When you walked into his house, there was human excrement on the floor. Cocaine is a powerful drug! People can't stop.

May 30, 1987   Cardwell C. Nuckols

Chapter 1

THE COCAINE EXPERIENCE

* A Drug for the 80's
  - More Than Euphoria
  - Dysfunctional Families
* Cocaine and Cultural Conditioning
* The Appeal of Cocaine
* Perceptions of Control
* Associating Sex and Cocaine
* Cocaine's Complex Effects
* Internal and External Cues
* Preconceptions
* The Setting
* The Effect of 'Cuts'
* Placebo Effects
* Side Effects

A well-known comedian I'll call Bill, recounts this conversation with a cocaine addict. He said, "Now why do you use that stuff? Can't you see that it's screwing up your life?" The person turned to him said, "But Bill, you know it intensifies your personality." Bill looks at him and says, "Yeah, but what if you're a jerk?"

Many people find *cocaine* a pleasant experience as long as they are around the people, places and things that reinforce the use of the drug, and no *adulterants* are in the drug that cause difficulty. A lot of people like to go to bars and use cocaine; others like to sit around the house and use it. Under these conditions cocaine produces intense pleasure sensations.

Among cocaine's nicer qualities is that it causes euphoria and general stimulation. In looking at the direct pharmacological effects of cocaine, you see that it shares attributes of the sexual act itself. When a person starts to become excited, what does cocaine do? On a biochemical level, it intensifies.

Cocaine does some profound things to the brain. In producing the perception of euphoria, it acts directly on the reward center of the brain. In 1954 James Olds investigated this center. He took electrodes and stimulated various areas of monkeys' brains. When precise areas of the brain were electrically stimulated, the monkey would get an erection or ejaculate without the presence of a female. All drugs that alter consciousness appear to act on this same part of the brain.

When you have a chemical that's behaviorally reinforcing because of its pleasurable action on the brain, what are the odds of using it again? There is nothing that gives a quicker emotional "turnaround" than cocaine. A pattern of repeated use arises when old behavioral reinforcement tells the brain there is no quicker way to feel good than to use cocaine.

Cocaine itself is an anesthetic, but it's a rare drug because it is also *sympathomimetic*. It mimics the effect of the sympathetic nervous system. The sympathetic nervous system is what triggers feelings of anxiousness and the fight-or-flight reaction for self-preservation. Have you ever been frightened? If you can, recall how you felt then. Fear is biomedically similar to someone "getting off" on cocaine.

There are parallels between the effects of cocaine and alcohol withdrawal. In a withdrawing alcoholic you see increased heart rate, enlarged pupils, increased blood pressure and psychomotor agitation. They are "all over the place." If you've ever watched the "down effects" of alcohol, you have a good idea of what the direct effects of cocaine intoxication are.

A DRUG FOR THE 80's

Cocaine has been available for a long time—over one hundred years. It was isolated in the 1850's or 1860's. Why have we chosen to use it excessively in the 1980's? When you talk to people who use cocaine and listen to their self-reports, cocaine's appeal is explained by citing its ability to produce euphoria. The energizing properties of the drug help overcome depression and *dysphoria*. It increases feelings of assertiveness, self-esteem, and frustration tolerance. It eliminates feelings of boredom and emptiness.

More Than Euphoria

I have concluded that there is more to the appeal of the drug than euphoria and its availability. I think it is no coincidence that when we started the breakdown of our families and the "do your own thing" movement, we began to see the emergence of a cocaine problem. Exhibitionism flourishes when people are high on cocaine; sexual exhibitionism and other types. Along with this came the compelling idea of entitlement. "I am entitled to freedom, stimulating experiences, and fulfillment." Cocaine magnifies this sense of entitlement. And, as is true with any chemical dependency, you see a deepening level of interpersonal exploitation. Cocaine causes us to exploit others in meeting what we perceive to be our own personal needs.

I've been impressed over the years by why people "do" the drugs they do. I started to look at why people selected cocaine in the late 70's, early 80's as the drug of choice. When I started to look back I noted that the decade of the 1950's was an interesting time in our country—a prosperous stable time. The early 1960's were still pleasant; things were very good for us. We had alcohol problems and some prescription drug problems, but on the whole it was a good time for our country.

As we reached the late 1960's and early 1970's, something started to happen that I think is still affecting us today. That something is the "me generation." We started to hear people like Timothy Leary say "drop out, tune in, turn on." We started to see an era of narcissism—to an extreme we'd never seen before. If we look at what society values and what emerged in this era of narcissism we will find data that speaks to the issues of why we look to cocaine for the peace that we think is missing inside us.

Dysfunctional Families

Looking around the country at people who are having cocaine-related difficulties, both children and adults, we see some revealing data. For example, I talked with a therapist, a psychologist from San Francisco named Kathleen O'Connell. She made the statement that in her private practice of twelve or thirteen years, ninety to ninety-five percent of all the cocaine addicts that she's treated came from dysfunctional homes, primarily homes where there was alcoholism.

Something happened to me recently, just a few weeks ago. This is a true story and I think it speaks to the heart of this issue, the problem of family values. I live in Chicago's Oak Forest area and have an office in Lombard, Illinois, close to the rich northwest suburbs of Chicago. One Sunday when I was getting ready to leave town I received a call from a perplexed mother who said, "You've just got to meet with our son. We think that he has a cocaine problem." I agreed that on my way to the airport I would stop and spend an hour with them—Mom, Dad, and son.

Soon after I got there Mom and Dad drove up in their brand new Cadillac. We sat there and talked for about fifteen minutes, waiting for Junior to show up. A very interesting thing happened: their son showed up in a $30,000 Porsche. I looked at Mom and Dad and said, "Did you buy this car for your son?" And they said, "No." I said, "Well, how did he get the money...to purchase this automobile?" They looked at each other, and Mom looked at Dad, and Dad looked back at Mom, and they looked at each other again...and suddenly Mom turned to me and said, " Well, I guess he must've got a part time job."

This is an atypical situation, but a dysfunctional family, nevertheless. I have personally treated cocaine *addiction* for ten years and have noticed the disproportionately large number of addicts coming from dysfunctional family backgrounds. Often, alcohol is involved. What does it mean to come from a dysfunctional family environment?

It means that your self-esteem is probably poor. Perhaps you don't know exactly who you are. Maybe your ego is not exactly what you would like it to be. Maybe you don't feel that you belong at times. The loaded question for this type of person is, "Who are you and what do you want? What do you do for fun?" These people often have a profound sense of isolation. Take this ego and self-esteem problem, this problem of identity and belonging, and remember it while we look at another related issue: cultural conditioning.

COCAINE AND CULTURAL CONDITIONING

Cocaine blends with the economics, politics, and social psychology of America in the 1980's like bathtub gin and the 1930's. Culturally conditioned aspirations, folk heroes and the hyperbole of advertising indirectly reinforce cocaine use even while it is officially condemned. Judgments about personal worth stress achievements, not who you are. Are you a vice-president? Do you own your own company? How much money do you make?

To illustrate the direction our culture shapes thought and behavior, consider, "When was the last time someone asked you about your spiritual program? When was the last time someone asked you about how good a parent you are? How good a husband? How good a wife? When was the last time someone asked you what we should do to change things back to a more pleasant way of life, when the family was the focus—before we started to see the disruption of the family and the problem of divorce and separation that we have today?"

For the masses, usually young, who lack and don't expect to achieve the glitter, cocaine is seductive. I recall conversations with cocaine users like this: "If you live in a neighborhood where everyone has Cadillacs, you have to have at least a BMW or Mercedes." A one-up social climate like this permeates the psychology and behavior of everyone. In a society that places so much emphasis on externals, on what you do and what you accomplish, a drug like cocaine creates a quick and dirty avenue for fulfilling human needs.

Ironically, it isn't just the person who doesn't achieve according to cultural ideals who becomes involved with cocaine, either. I've counseled people who are cocaine dependent even though super-successes by cultural standards. In male cocaine addicts we often see family heroes, people who judge themselves and are judged by what they do in the world of work. These people are out there hustling. Inside they feel empty. For these victims of their own success, cocaine fulfills a missing sense of importance and boosts feelings of self-worth. Preoccupied with the fantasy of unlimited success, power, brilliance, beauty or ideal love, they embrace cocaine. What is missing is that internal peace, that internal gratification, that internal reward.

Take these two extremes, the external priorities of our society and the numbers of people with perceived internal deficits, and add something that brings these two realms together to make a whole. That something is cocaine. Cocaine is a drug that enhances one's sense of ego. It creates the illusion of belonging—it is a power and control drug for people who are hustling in the fast lane, but on the inside still don't feel like they belong. They don't feel like they're everything in the world they want to be. But when you put cocaine in there, suddenly there's a feeling of wholeness. Cocaine provides a sense of power, potency and control that they may not have perceived before. This is the common denominator of the drug of choice of the 1980's.

THE APPEAL OF COCAINE

To appreciate the appeal of cocaine to the adolescent or young adult exposed to today's social pressures, consider an advertisement for a cocaine treatment program. On one side of the brochure is a list of the properties of cocaine, and on the other side, a list of the problems that cocaine causes. You read the properties of cocaine and see that it makes you feel alert. It causes you to lose your appetite so it makes you slim and trim. People will love you because it causes you to talk a lot. ("I'm shy and have trouble going out and meeting people.") Besides all these things, cocaine causes you to feel euphoric. "I'm not going to read the other side of the brochure, because I know that this must be the drug for me."

If you think about this, in the 80's, these are the important things to have. We want to be trim. We want to be the life of the party. We want to be out there and be involved. Cocaine helps meet these needs.

PERCEPTIONS OF CONTROL

What is a person's subjective experience when they *snort* a couple of lines of cocaine? If you think about two people who sit down and snort cocaine and talk to one another, its almost as if they met every criteria for the diagnosis: *narcissistic personality disorder.* They have an exaggerated sense of self-importance. The universe revolves around them. They adopt the posture of important people. If you have low self-esteem or if you're vulnerable to power and control urges, cocaine is the drug for you.

People with poor self-esteem, stressed and bored, have a high incidence of cocaine use. To augment a hyperactive, restless lifestyle and the need for self-sufficiency, people use cocaine. Like every drug I've known, whether a depressant or stimulant, cocaine gives the feeling that you're in control. Paradoxically, cocaine is a profound central nervous system stimulant. When someone uses it you'd think it would make them rattle a little. But most people describe an enhanced sense of internal control when using cocaine.

ASSOCIATING SEX AND COCAINE

If you've been around addicts you've heard some of the things they talk about. One thing that's prominent is the association between sex and cocaine. Many people see cocaine as an aphrodisiac. At low doses the male can maintain an erection for hours. They aren't orgasmic.

However, if two regular sex partners are frequent cocaine users, the quality of their relationship is affected by the drug. There's emotional distancing in the relationship. Probably the only thing they're giving each other in the relationship is cocaine. They probably have poor communication and have never looked each other in the eye. Who would want to look at someone with cocaine eyes anyway? They aren't a pretty sight to see.

As cocaine use accelerates, males lose the ability to have an erection. You lose the ability to have an orgasm. And you start to get *kinky* to compensate for your lost sexual performance. Some of the stories told by everyday middle class Americans using cocaine sound like scripts for X-rated movies. People who preferred "man on top, get it over quick" are now "into" sado-masochism and bondage. The behavioral alterations, the physiological and psychological changes produced by cocaine are profound.

COCAINE'S COMPLEX EFFECTS

When you try to generalize about the effects of cocaine, whether administered *intravenously, intranasally,* or smoked as *freebase,* you must consider several things beyond the drug itself. For example, if you are talking about total drug effect, there are many sub-populations of users. This is true for any substance of abuse. Some people experience intense anxiety from just one marijuana cigarette. Many things combine to create a drug's effect. A complex set of interactions influence one's response to cocaine: 1) the direct pharmacological effect of the drug; 2) the effects of *cuts* or adulterants added to the drug; 3) the personality of the user; and 4) the physical and social environment.

INTERNAL AND EXTERNAL CUES

Among the most important sources of cocaine's effect are the *internal* and *external cues* associated with its use. Internal cues are represented by the psychological make-up of the individual. Internal cues include the person's perception, past experience, expectations, and all the biochemical events occurring in the body. Internal cues include how a person feels today. Are you sick? Have you eaten well?

External cues are primarily what may be called the people, places and things. Things are money in the pocket, Eric Clapton's cocaine song on the radio—different sorts of cues associated with using cocaine.

PRECONCEPTIONS

What if someone told you that they had done cocaine and turned into a raving monster? Your perception might be that if I take cocaine I will have a negative reaction. This beforehand perception of the event may cause you to have an unsatisfactory, distressing experience. In contrast, if someone told you, "Cocaine is the most marvelous drug you'll ever do in your life. Do a couple of lines of cocaine and you'll be in heaven," your perception of the drug's effect would be different.

THE SETTING

Consider the *setting* for cocaine use. You are out in the world of people, places and things, and you are out "doing some cocaine." In contrast, let's say that you are in a sterile white laboratory where a technician is administering cocaine. Your experience will be different. Probably the anxiety that cocaine can cause will be in the forefront. If you are in a situation where the external cue is a beautiful woman in a dimly lit setting, offering cocaine as a precursor to sexual intercourse, you will have a different drug experience than in the laboratory. *Set* and setting are important determinants of your drug experience.

THE EFFECT OF 'CUTS' (Adulterants)

Drug effects are often mediated by some of the cuts or adulterants that are used to extend or dilute the substance. If a cocaine user says he took one *toot* and went directly to the bathroom, what he is possibly telling you is that the cocaine was cut with a baby laxative called *monito*. Monito is a cut that looks good. Its white crystalline flakes look just like the drug itself and it has little effect of its own.

What else is used as cut in street cocaine? What adulterants are used? At the time of this writing, street cocaine has become very potent, and is getting stronger. Cuts that are popular today are sugars such as *manatol* and *inositol*. Cocaine is also cut with *lidocaine, procaine, carbacaine,* or any of the 'caines.' These are all anesthetics which give you that *freeze* that mimics the direct anesthetic effect of cocaine.

PLACEBO EFFECTS

There are other substances on the street that mimic the effect of cocaine. Have you ever read a *head magazine,* where you see mail order ads for white crystalline powders that you can stuff up your nose? It's not cocaine and not illegal. They're the "look-a-likes." We've had the look-a-like amphetamines; the little black biphetamine, "black beauty," sold through stores somewhat legitimately. Well, the same thing is happening with cocaine. There have been some studies showing that people who use cocaine can actually "get off" on the *placebo effect.*

Although cocaine is a powerful drug, the placebo effect can be taken advantage of. If you went out tonight and bought one hundred dollars worth of something that was junk, you'd "get off" on it. That is the placebo effect. You'll find it over and over again. Often, experienced users can't tell the difference between cocaine and lidocaine, perhaps a primary component of the gram they just bought.

SIDE EFFECTS

Cocaine has some side effects that are discouraging. It causes you to grate your teeth and get all tight. You sometimes see almost a heroin-type syndrome when you have a person come into treatment saying their muscles hurt. You say to yourself "That is not what cocaine withdrawal is supposed to look like." But it's what it looks like if you've been tight for two days. When you're all hunched over and tight, once those muscles start to relax, they get very tender and sore. Side effects are why high-dose users display a common pattern. The uncomfortable side effects of cocaine are edginess, anxiety, and paranoia. In reaction, high-dose users will begin using central nervous system depressants to "take the *edge* off," to take a little of the *crank* off the drug.

It's becoming common to see paranoid responses among high-dose cocaine users. They run to the window every time a car goes by to see it is the police. Then they begin using other drugs to help *titrate* the dysphoric effects of the cocaine.

Unless a person has another psychiatric problem, their paranoia will be an exaggeration of their immediate fears. If they are a street dealer they are going to think that the *narcs* are in the closet. If they've been "ripping off" their company and they work for the Chicago Board of Trade, they're going to be afraid the IRS is in the closet. Their paranoia is an exaggeration of a normal and understandable fear, magnified and continuous. So the most common thing you'll notice in a behavioral profile of a cocaine addict is escalation. Besides more and more cocaine, they will use alcohol and pot. This is your typical profile. Often you'll see other central nervous system depressants used such as *quaaludes*. Mainly you'll see valium, librium, and other tranquilizers and sleeping pills—any form of central nervous system depressant.

Chapter 2

COCAINE: THE DRUG

COCAINE'S ORIGINS

Cocaine is an illegal drug, smuggled into the United States primarily from South America. The coca plant, whose leaves supply the drug, requires high altitudes to grow. Soil, altitude and climatic conditions in the Andes mountains of South America are ideal for cocaine horticulture. Recently, however, we've begun to see some attempts at growing the coca plant in the United States. In 1985, coca plants were discovered growing on the Hawaiian Islands and arrests were made.

Cocaine is considered a "Schedule II" drug by the United States federal government. A Schedule II drug is one with high potential for abuse having legitimate medical uses. First offense penalties for trafficking in cocaine range from five to fifteen years in prison and a fifteen to twenty-five thousand dollar fine. Appendix A contains an overview of the *Controlled Substances Act of 1970* which governs federal drug penalties.

In the mountains of South America, cocaine provided a service to the Indians for generations. Native Indians worked long hours at high altitudes with little food. By chewing the coca leaves, as some Americans chew tobacco, appetites were reduced. The absorption of the drug through the mucous membrane provided an energizing effect. Chewing the coca leaf made them feel more like working and not eating. These attributes were important among people who worked long hours in the mountain air with low oxygen content. To them, coca leaves were a blessing, a gift from the Sun God.

PRODUCING COCAINE HYDROCHLORIDE

In the mid-1800's we discovered how to isolate a potent, crystalline, white powder from the coca leaf. The coca leaf in its natural form is about one percent cocaine, but we learned how to refine the leaf material into a ninety-nine percent pure white powder. We learned that the powder could be introduced into our bodies by injecting it as a solution or by *snorting* it through the nose. We discovered that if we injected a cocaine solution, the drug would reach our brain in about fourteen seconds. If snorted, it would get there in about three to four minutes. If we chewed it, fifteen or twenty minutes would elapse before an effect was felt. That effect was mild, like coffee.

Looking at the source of cocaine, the coca bush, about one percent of the leaf's weight comprises its active ingredient. Cocaine is found naturally in a form called an alkaloid.

Alkaloid means 'something like' an alkaline substance. (On some Mondays we're 'humanoids'—more or less human). As an alkaline-like substance, cocaine has a high *pH* index.

The problem with alkaloidal cocaine is that if you try to snort or inject it, about a quart of water is required to dissolve one gram. To inject alkaloidal cocaine, you'd need a syringe big enough to hold a quart of water. You'd probably die of over-hydration before you could get the drug into your system. This is impractical. Snorting alkaloidal cocaine would be like packing mud up your nose. It wouldn't dissolve well.

So, modern chemistry is applied. From basic chemistry we know that if you add an acid, in this case hydrochloric acid, to an alkaloid, we get a salt— *cocaine hydrochloride.* Cocaine hydrochloride is highly water soluble. You can take ten or twelve drops of water, put them in a gram of cocaine hydrochloride, and have a perfectly clear solution.

Most of the cocaine that has been smuggled into the United States during recent years has been in the form of cocaine hydrochloride, processed in the kitchens of Peru, Equador, Bolivia or Columbia. Cocaine hydrochloride is suitable for snorting or injecting, but we still have a problem. It's difficult to smoke, the fastest and most direct method of getting a drug to the brain.

HOW COCAINE IS ADMINISTERED

Few people take or "drop" cocaine orally. We can't digest it and pass it into our systems efficiently, like food. It works poorly that way. The acids in the stomach don't degrade the cocaine, but the "high impact" potency of the drug is virtually lost. Also, oral administration produces a slow onset of effect. There would be no *rush,* the experience sought by cocaine users.

Intranasal Administration

The most common way of administering cocaine is by the intra-nasal route. It takes the drug three to four minutes to get from nose to brain. It must first penetrate the mucous membrane, a rate-limiting step. It must dissolve in water, get into the mucous membrane, go into the veins, the *vena cava*, the right side of the heart, then be pumped through the lungs to the left side of the heart and out to the brain and body. Additional time is required for the drug to get into the brain and produce an effect.

Injection

When you inject cocaine into your arm with a hypodermic syringe, what happens is a little different. The same basic route comes into play, but the cocaine travels from arm to brain in about fourteen seconds. It goes into the veins, the vena cava, the right side of the heart, the lungs, again the left heart and up into the brain.

I once thought that the most economical way to get any drug into the system was to inject it. I also thought that injecting was the most dangerous way to get drugs into the system. With *freebasing*, which I'll describe later, neither statement is true.

People who injected cocaine, back in the late 1960's and early 1970's, would inject half of their cocaine, wait a few seconds and see if "the bells came out." Are you familiar with a sixties dance called the "hucklebuck?" When people become toxic from cocaine and start getting close to overdose, they start doing the hucklebuck. You can't hear; you start *strobing*. You can't see, and your body starts to shake.

I was talking to a man and we were comparing war stories. He said, "You know, when I started to get the hucklebuck, when I was *shooting up* in the early seventies, that was the point I wanted to be at. I always had to be careful when I got that toxic because I didn't want to give myself too much. So I would put half the cocaine in and wait a little while. When I started to shake, if I could still get the other half in I would put it in. If I couldn't, just from my arm motion, I would usually throw the syringe across the room. Then I would always be on the floor. There would be a moment of truth. I wanted to know if it was the room shaking or me shaking. So I had a little mirror that I put right down on floor level. And I would look over there and see that, yes, it was me doing the hucklebuck, and yes, it was where I wanted to be."

That is bordering on *seizure;* bordering on extreme overdose. That's the crazy thrill and rush. That's where people can get when they're injecting cocaine. You can't get to that point snorting cocaine up your nose. You may get fifty, one hundred, or two hundred *nanogram percent* blood levels from putting it up your nose. But you are talking one thousand to twelve hundred nanogram percent blood level from injecting and freebasing.

Freebasing

Smoking cocaine results in acutely high blood levels of the drug. When a person freebases, inhales cocaine vapors into their lungs, in only six to eight seconds cocaine is hitting the brain. It by-passes the right side of heart and lungs and goes straight to the left heart and out to the brain. Freebase is rapidly increasing in popularity. Many people start out using cocaine intranasally and then progress to freebasing. However, with recent changes in the packaging and distribution of cocaine, many youth now begin their involvement with cocaine by smoking it in the form of *rock* or *crack.*

Cocaine has been smoked in South America for years in the form of coca paste, a cocaine sulfate. We called it base. In South America, the paste smoked is about thirty percent cocaine. Nevertheless, smoking paste is now the leading cause of psychiatric admission in Columbia.

Cocaine in its base form, right out of the coca plant, is more the alkaloid or pure product. You heat it to a lower temperature to vaporize it. In other words, it is more volatile than cocaine hydrochloride. With cocaine in its base form, you are getting about fifty percent of the cocaine into the system with a good pipe.

Converting Cocaine Hydrochloride

The main import into this country, however, is cocaine hydro-chloride. To smoke the cocaine that is available we had to find a way to change its characteristics, to "convert" it. One of the things you'll find in chemistry books is that it takes intense heat to make cocaine hydrochloride, a very stable compound, go from a solid, flaky, white material into a gas—a process termed *sublimation.* It requires a temperature of approximately 359 degrees Fahrenheit. At this high temperature, much of the cocaine is destroyed.

To avoid destroying the costly drug, it is better to convert the cocaine hydrochloride back into its alkaloid form. In its alkaloid form, cocaine will vaporize at approximately 209 degrees Fahrenheit. We've found many creative ways to make this conversion. One way to think about freebase is to look at the equation or formula for cocaine hydrochloride, and imagine freeing the alkaloidal cocaine from the hydrochloride salt. This returns the substance to its original alkaloid form that will vaporize at only 209 degrees. Most of the cocaine is retained during the conversion and the end product will produce that euphoric, eight-second rush when smoked.

The terms we hear on the street for freebase are rock or crack. I first heard the term rock in the Oakland/Los Angeles area. The term crack seems to have arisen from the cracking sound that freebase cocaine makes when you *"torch* it," or heat it, so it goes from a solid state to a gaseous state for inhalation.

The old way of making this conversion was the Richard Pryor method, using ether.   The problem with ether is that it is flammable. Ether is also heavier than air and dissipates slowly. If you put a can of ether on the table, its vapors will fall and creep along the floor. And it takes a lot of minutes for your area to ventilate enough to light a match safely. Richard Pryor talks about his freebase experience, where he set himself on fire. The accident happened while trying to light a freebase pipe with ether still in the air. This story, however, has changed over time. Richard now describes the event as a suicide attempt, possibly related to his use of freebase.

The federal government has started to regulate the sales of ether, so it is not as readily available now as it once was. But we found we could use other ubiquitous solvents to make the conversion. For example you could take things right out of mom's pantry, like baking soda, or go into the laundry room and get ammonia bleach, or ammonia.

Baking soda or ammonia can be used to reverse the equation I mentioned earlier, taking cocaine hydrochloride back to the alkaloid. We invented a simple conversion process called *"shake and bake."* One way to do this is to get a little plastic container, put in the cocaine hydrochloride dissolved in water, add ammonia, shake it up, and use a double boiler or other heat source to catalyze the reaction. What precipitates, or coagulates, is the alkaloidal form of cocaine. This is dried out and sold in little hunks or rocks, or in larger rectangular shapes called *slabs.*

I was sitting in my office with a mother and her fifteen and sixteen year old adolescent children. She was concerned about her children, drugs, all the strange friends they were hanging around, their school performance, and that things were just not going well for the family. She described all these problems and finally said, "... and on top of that, both of my kids got microwaves and none of them cook in their rooms." Well, the kids were using the microwaves for the heat catalyzation of this reaction, a process known as *"nuking* the cocaine." So the kids were nuking the cocaine. And when mom said that, both the kids almost crawled under their chairs. I mean they knew it was "up"—they'd been exposed. They were both using microwave ovens to catalyze the reaction and rapidly dry the cocaine for smoking.

Manufacturing smokeable cocaine has become less hazardous in terms of not having to worry about blowing yourself up. There are even kits that can be purchased with solvents in them. These kits, bought at "head" shops or through the mail, produce base cocaine with a purity as high as ninety-five to ninety-seven and one-half percent. People are dying from it because it is so potent. We are seeing two hundred to three hundred percent increases in overdoses in major urban areas across the country from freebase.

Smoking Cocaine

A water pipe is the instrument most often used to smoke cocaine—the same type of water pipe that came out of the 60's with the marijuana culture. There is liquid in the pipe and a little receptacle for the cocaine. You use a *torch* to light it. The torch can be a lighter or a match, or sometimes a coat hanger and a little piece of cotton ball soaked in 151 proof rum. The cocaine vapor is sucked in through the pipe, through the liquid. The liquid may be wine, it may be Corvoissier cognac, it may be 151 proof rum (depending upon your preference). You inhale this gas directly into your mouth and lungs.

Another way of freebasing is to simply use a straight, heat resistant tube. People put the rock in the tube, heat it, and inhale the gases directly into the lungs. Straight pipe users should worry about possible lung damage. With the water pipe you have a cooling system and a filtration system. With the straight pipe you're getting nothing but a straight, unfiltered, hot gas into our lungs and throat. These organs are unsuited for handling that intense heat.

Hazards of Freebasing

There are several physical hazards to smoking cocaine. We know from the Len Bias story that cocaine can kill. We know that some people display violent physical reactions to cocaine and can die the first time they use it. We know that other people will have changes in their tolerance to the drug, a process we call *kindling*. Kindling is a form of reverse tolerance where from one week to the next people may not know how well they will tolerate their customary levels of cocaine use.

Experts seem to agree that if someone continues to inhale a hot gas with all sorts of breakdown products into their lungs, early chronic obstructive lung disease is likely to occur. We may see the early onset of emphysema in some of the adolescents and young adults who are starting to use rock and crack cocaine.

Another problem has been brought to my attention. I had the opportunity to talk with a toxicologist and medical examiner from the Miami area. One of the people, Dr. Wetli, mentioned that upon autopsy, he was seeing adolescents whose coronary arteries looked like they were fifty to sixty years old. He said the process of smoking cocaine can cause a narrowing of the coronary arteries. Injecting cocaine may produce similar damage. It may be transient narrowing, but somehow the body is interpreting it as damage. The linings of the inside of those arteries are getting more and more occluded. We expect to see some cardiovascular problems arising at an early age in the cocaine-using population.

People who freebase or use cocaine intravenously *(I.V.)* are usually more out of control. Although you have people who intranasally use large amounts of the drug, the severity of its impact on the central nervous system, compared with freebase and I.V., is less profound. You cannot assimilate enough cocaine through snorting to match the blood levels in the brain you get from freebase and I.V.

For example, if you go out and snort a few grams or an *eight-ball* (eighth of an *ounce*), you may achieve a blood level of two hundred to four hundred nanogram percent. That is the peak. If you go out and freebase a quarter of an ounce, or an ounce, you could display one thousand to twelve hundred nanogram percent blood level. This is an increase of three to six times the blood level of the drug. Therefore, you infer that there is significant impact on the brain's thought and emotional processes. There may be greater distortion. I also think that the lifestyles of people who use cocaine intraveneously, or who freebase, become radically different from social snorters'.

MARKETING COCAINE TO YOUTH

We notice that it was the post-World War II baby boom generation, people now in their thirties and forties, who introduced cocaine in the 1960's and 1970's. They were the primary consumers. But like the heroin addict who *matures out* in his middle to late thirties, we started to see some maturing

out of middle-aged, cocaine-addicted individuals. Thus, the
market for cocaine began to flatten out in terms of escalating
numbers.

If we were involved in the business of making money from
cocaine we might think, "What population of people could we
sell cocaine to, making a better buck?" Well, I think it's
obvious. We have a brand new consumer line right now, a
product that hits quick—freebase—and we can develop that and
sell it to a young market. To sell it to a young market we do
exactly what pharmaceutical companies do: *unit dose* it.

Unit Dosing Crack and Rock Cocaine

Crack and rock cocaine, or freebase cocaine, is marketed to a
younger population. The targeted market is youth ranging in
age from twelve years to their twenty's. These are the primary
consumers of crack and rock, the market the product is
designed for. Unit dosing has brought price structure changes
that make cocaine available even to youth with limited funds.
Five or ten years ago, if we wanted to go out and "party like
crazy and grab some cocaine," we had to come up with about
one hundred dollars for a gram. If I was fifteen years old and
I had one hundred dollars in my pocket (which is highly
unlikely), I would face a big choice. I could drink for a month
or more. Or, I could smoke *reefer* for a month. But to spend
one hundred dollars on a white substance I've never tried, and
that would only last for an evening—that was an unlikely
choice. Also, the purity of the product was poor, and we
looked at cocaine as a narcotic—a street drug.

With a one-unit dose of rock or crack cocaine costing as little
as two-fifty, no higher than ten dollars, cocaine becomes
attractive to youth. At these prices, crack or rock is within
their financial means. Incidentally, on the surface it appears
that crack cocaine is cheap. Crack cocaine is no cheaper than
snorting cocaine. You will pay a fractional, proportionate price
of bulk cocaine. You see, it takes several rocks, perhaps ten,
to make a gram (depending on the size of the rocks), and at
ten dollars a rock you're still paying one hundred dollars a
gram. These figures change according to the "going price" of

cocaine but the relationship remains stable. It's not cheaper, it just appears cheaper. In the long run it will be more expensive because of the high doses that people use in their love affair with cocaine.

In terms of product lines coming into this country, we're seeing an influx of pre-processed crack or rock. We know, for example, that just about the only product line you can get through the Bahamas is rock or crack: freebaseable, smokeable cocaine. Often we're seeing home laboratories or small "set-ups" that take cocaine hydrochloride and convert it—a new "cottage industry."

THE COCAINE GLUT

Cocaine prices obey the economic laws of supply and demand. The street price of cocaine averages between sixty and one hundred dollars per gram at the time of this writing. In rural Ohio you may still have to pay one hundred dollars or more to *score* a gram of cocaine, while in Miami, Florida you can get cocaine in gram portions, that may be as high as seventy to ninety percent pure, for fifty to sixty dollars. Right now it's a buyer's market. Everyone is saying that the cocaine glut is just starting. With a cocaine glut, prices are down and quality is up.

ADULTERANTS

A few years ago when you saw crack cocaine or a base rock, you could be sure it was pure, without adulterants. But now we're starting to see quality control problems in rock and crack cocaine. You don't know what's in it. You can find all sorts of things in there. We're seeing cuts in rock and crack. These are techniques for expanding weight and volume and adding other drugs for impact. For example, some people have been adding drain cleaner to rock and crack processing to increase weight, volume and profits. If you look at what the adolescent consumer buys, the powdered type of the drug is still hit-and-miss. Often it isn't cocaine. It could be several different things from *PCP* to caffeine, to a little *amphetamine,* to nothing more than just an inert white powder. When we see rock or crack, however, it is usually purer. But there is the growing potential of added adulterants.

POLYDRUGS

The product line is changing, too. Combinations of drugs are being sold to cocaine users, complicating the addiction picture. Rock and crack are not only unit-dosed but are sometimes sold in what is called a "slab." You can buy three or four different *hits* in a slab. A slab may be pure cocaine, ninety-seven percent, or it could be cut with PCP (called *space base*), or heroin (like a *speedball* used in the heroin culture).

Sometimes these drug combinations, for example the classic "speedball," are designed to minimize a particular side effect. The classic speedball is cocaine with heroin, usually injected. Today it's a buyer's market and sellers are sensitive to the types of drugs people want. There are sophisticated marketing schemes.

In Miami, for instance, someone said, "Look, we had a big report that said cocaine causes a reduction in vitamins B and C." We soon began to pick up cocaine that was laced with vitamins B and C. Another paper came out that said people who snort cocaine end up with sinus infections; there was bacteria in the cocaine. Soon, cases turned up where people came into emergency rooms with an allergic reaction to the penicillin found in their cocaine.

Chapter 3

COCAINE DEPENDENCE

* Rapid Addiction
* A Unique Progression
* Cocaine Anguish
* What About Recreational Cocaine Use?
* The Addictive Process
* Personality, Temperament and Addiction
* Compulsive Use as Self-Medication
* The Role of Childhood Hyperkinesia
* The Polydrug Complication
    - Unawareness of Complete Drug Use Pattern
* Psychiatric Disorders
    - Depression
* Instant Gratification

Andrew Wiel, in *Chocolate to Morphine,* says there is nothing wrong with drugs. They are neither inherently good nor bad. People use them for reasons that often lead to serious problems, creating bad relationships between the consumer and the drug. Tragically, that appears to be the norm with cocaine.

I was in Connecticut lecturing on cocaine, intimacy, and sexual relationships. I noticed a lady in the audience crying. During the break I took her aside and said, "What happened? It seems there's something occurring in your life related to what we're talking about." She said, "Yes, my husband is a doctor and he just picked cocaine over me. We're getting a divorce."

I hear this a lot. "Cocaine can't hug me or kiss me; it can't give me affection. Yet I will pick this damn white substance over people who can do nice things for me in the world. I pick it over my job. Pick it over anything. Half of the time, I pick it over sex—but I would prefer to have sex with it."

RAPID ADDICTION

With cocaine addiction, we're simply saying "this person can't stop." I've often asked patients who were cocaine addicts, "What do you think about this stuff? Do you think it causes physical dependency?" The reply has generally been, "I used to think cocaine wasn't physically addictive but when, for the thousandth time, I tried but couldn't stop using it, I figured I had a problem. Maybe I was dependent."

When you ask people who use cocaine regularly if they have a dependency problem, what you hear is "Yes, I do, because I can't stop. Even when I want to stop, I can't stop. Nine out of ten times I can't refuse cocaine. Nine out of ten times, even when I don't want to use cocaine, just being physically close to it causes me to use again. If I take one line, I'll take every bit I can get my hands on. I may even start calling people at 4 A.M."

A UNIQUE PROGRESSION

Alcohol and cocaine dependents share the same patterns of initial reactions to the drug experience. Cocaine dependents often say, "I remember a time when I thought I could never do more than a half or one gram of cocaine a night." Then there are those who are captivated, who "get down" in their first episode. With cocaine, however, the progression of the drug dependency is different than with alcohol.

An alcoholic may spend from five to thirty years developing the addiction we call alcoholism; all the psychological, behavioral, social, spiritual problems of chemical dependency.

With adolescents freebasing cocaine, we see a progression to a situation requiring intensive treatment in from two to six months. With adults, we're seeing anywhere from six months to three or four years of heavy use, to develop the same levels and types of difficulties it takes twenty years for chronic alcoholics to develop.

Dr. Doug Talbot, a well known *addictionologist*, believes there is a drug dependency progression that occurs within the brain itself. When a person starts using drugs, conscious choice governs. The cerebral cortex, the computer part of the brain, enables this person to turn off their drug use early, get to bed, and do the things they need to do. But as drug use continues, something happens so that the person becomes dependent upon the chemical, physiologically and psychologically.

Dr. Talbot believes that what happens is that at some point the drug takes on a property that the brain interprets as an instinct, something necessary for survival. In watching my father die of alcoholism and watching others die of addiction, his is the only explanation that makes sense to me. The drug's having taken on an instinctive quality equated with survival is the only way I can explain the behaviors I see among cocaine addicts.

Related to the inability to stop is the inability to conserve the drug, to put some away for tomorrow. This is also sometimes true of people who have become dependent upon marijuana, heroin, alcohol, tranquilizers, sedatives, and the "Heinz 57" variety of drugs that alter consciousness. Why is it that when people become chemically dependent they can't leave a little bit for tomorrow? It's rare to find a cocaine addict who is going to save any at all. They say things like this to themselves: "I have two grams left and I want to put some of it away." They can't bring themselves to do it though. The anguish of coming off this drug and the strong components of addiction that are involved in using cocaine make it practically impossible.

COCAINE ANGUISH

The *Diagnostic and Statistical Manual* of the American Psychiatric Association (*The DSM-III*) declares cocaine abstinence a disorder that induces people to use cocaine. The dysphoria or anguish of coming off cocaine is profound. When you are getting off a drug like alcohol, you are *coming down* for several hours. Distributing the experience of coming down over several hours doesn't seem to result in the intense anguish of cocaine abstinence. Cocaine "takes you up" quickly, but drops you fast too. If it hits your brain within six to eight seconds, in the time it takes to get the freebase pipe from your mouth to the table, you experience a "coming down" that is precipitous.

Coming off cocaine is one of the most anguished, depressing experiences. I've watched people talk about coming off freebase and one of the things that I noticed was the non-verbal maneuvers used to describe it. It appears like they're describing a heart attack. They have fists clenched to the chest. You can see that it hurts. They can recreate that hurt for you because it's a devastating event. You'll do almost anything to keep from *crashing* on cocaine. And on top of that you'll do just about anything to keep your supply coming. Post-cocaine anguish is a strong inducement to use again—to keep the pain away.

WHAT ABOUT RECREATIONAL COCAINE USE?

There are moral and legal issues pertaining to using cocaine. It is an illegal drug. These raise serious questions about the notion "recreational use" of cocaine. From a clinical perspective it is difficult to answer the question, "What is recreational cocaine use?" Are there people who can use cocaine without experiencing trouble with it? There may be a sub-population of people who can "do a little bit" of cocaine, put it away, "do a little bit more later," and not have problems. But therapists and counselors don't have people coming to them saying, "I snorted two lines of cocaine last night. Can you help me? I enjoyed the hell out of it." The people may be out there somewhere but they aren't part of the clinical scene yet. The cocaine users therapists and counselors see are those who have lost families, health, jobs and hope. They are victims of a progressive addiction.

THE ADDICTIVE PROCESS

Unfortunately, some of the basic reference materials used by psychologists, psychiatrists and other clinicians, for example the *DSM-III* mentioned earlier, describe cocaine as a substance of abuse—but not a substance of *dependence*. The notion is that you can distinguish between the mind and the body, and that the crucial issue is what happens to the body. Dependence is a physical phenomenon. But I don't think you can differentiate the mind from the body. In terms of consequences for the drug user, his family and the community, what difference does it make if his destruction has arisen from a psychological abuse (mind) or a physical dependence (body)? The truth is, he can't stop using cocaine and is in desperate trouble.

I have worked with people who have used cocaine for less than a year and whose lives were already shattered. One gentleman in particular comes to mind. In nine months he had blown $150,000, had lost his whole family, owed another $50,000, and was in an auto wreck. He had blown everything...from job to family. The progressive nature of the illness is astonishing.

I am convinced, from my work with drug users, that cocaine causes both psychological and physiological dependence just as alcohol, valium and many other drugs do. We see consistent patterns of *electroencephalogram* changes, bio-chemical changes, and repeatedly observe the same set of symptoms in early recovery. These facts tell me that cocaine is a physical dependency-causing chemical.

PERSONALITY, TEMPERAMENT AND ADDICTION

Your personality and temperament are a major influence on your choice of drugs and how you use them. *With or without drugs,* I've found that people repeat the behaviors that produce the neural transmissions they want to feel. For me, lecturing produces some of the same excitement and thrill that cocaine did. So I choose to do it. Think about it. I started to lecture about ten years ago, within a few years of giving up cocaine. Lecturing remains a thrilling experience. I get that anticipatory excitement before I come out to speak to a group. I love it. I crave it. I don't think I will ever change. I don't think I will ever be a person who doesn't like stimulation.

I know of no technique that will let me take a cocaine person, who loves excitement, and say, "Okay, now you don't like excitement any more. Now you just want to be middle-of-the-road. You don't like the cutting edge anymore. Just put that in your mind." It just doesn't work. So what I have to start thinking of is that I want that cocaine dependent to experience excitement, but I want it to be appropriate. I want him to get his thrills in ways that do not result in problems.

With the woman's husband who chose cocaine over her, we have a physician who found, through experimentation, a chemical and a set of behaviors that met a perceived need. Are there any general statements or rules that apply here? I think so. However, no general system that tries to explain drug-related behavior fits every case. You can usually come up with cases that challenge any system. Nevertheless, I have found it useful to consider people's coping-styles and how they "tie into" drug use patterns. I have been impressed by the consistent relationships between coping-style and gravitation to stimulants or depressants.

People who use central nervous system depressants—alcohol, opiates, tranquilizers, sleeping pills, and pot—tend to cope with stress through isolation and relaxation. It's more an avoidance dynamic. It is a "take in to keep down." What do depressants do? They reduce neural transmissions in the brain. Take a person functioning at his typical level. If he wants to shut out internal dialogue or "chatter in the head," wants to shut out a lot of stimulation, consider the effect of two or three ten milligram valiums and a shot of heroin. It reduces the number of neural transmissions in the brain. He won't be thinking about much because there won't be "a whole lot of neural firing there." People who want to go on a true honeymoon and end up in a vacuum, "*shoot* heroin." They think about nothing then.

I find that people who use stimulant drugs want to confront a hostile environment with intellectual or physical activity. It is more of an arousal model. They need to be in control. They need to be on the cutting edge. They need to be able to "deal with" the situation. I find that they jump in, both feet first, even when they don't know what they're doing. These are the general differences I see between people who use depressants and stimulants.

COMPULSIVE USE AS SELF-MEDICATION

I believe that compulsive use of a chemical can often be seen as an attempt at self-medication. Every client I've seen, even if they were psychotic, sought and usually found a drug to help them deal with their problems. People learn what to take in to make themselves feel better. We find that people learn how to self-medicate. To understand how people function as their own pharmacologists, Andrew Wiel's book, *The Natural Mind,* is an excellent resource. *Finding the drug that works for us isn't a random process.* We search until we find one that provides the relief we seek.

Drugs can help us cope with a feeling or a problem—people, places and things that we don't handle well. Whenever I talk to someone about their chemical dependency I ask, "What did you get out of this drug? What is the good part of it?" "Oh, it made me feel good. It made me feel like I was one of the crowd. When I had cocaine in my pocket all the chicks really dug me. I always had a lot of friends, and before that I was always a very lonely person." Anyone who wants to help the person with a drug problem must listen carefully to the answers to these questions.

The drug user is getting something from the drug that is perceived as valuable. I have observed that clients prefer drugs that help them cope with the feelings that trouble them the most. I think that to a great degree the "feeling" problems dictate drug choice more than the "people, places, and things" problems. People experiment with a whole range of drugs to find the one that best suits their own unique psychological needs.

THE ROLE OF CHILDHOOD HYPERKINESIA

There is a relationship between childhood *hyperkinesia* and the use of cocaine as an adult. There may also may be a correation between childhood attention deficits and later cocaine use. If you've ever sat down and looked at the toxin-induced hypervigilance of a cocaine user, it's almost like being in a Ping-Pong match. It's difficult to talk with someone who is high on cocaine because with every little sound they react. A person who is high on cocaine lacks the ability to focus his attention and maintain it. There is some research that shows that the auditory acuity of cocaine users is higher than the general population's.

THE POLYDRUG COMPLICATION

People who work with clients in chemical dependency programs believe in abstinence from all drugs. However, in dealing with cocaine dependence we often hear clients claim that cocaine is the only chemical they've had trouble with. While they may perceive cocaine as undesirable and a source of extreme problems, they don't want to forego the other drugs they use. They say, "Cocaine is the only thing I ever lost control over in my whole life. You see, I've been drinking for ten years and smoking pot for fifteen years. I never had a problem with that. So don't tell me I'm going to have to give that up, too."

That is the first hurdle in the struggle to help the cocaine addict recover from his illness. Do we keep the cocaine dependent in treatment even while he uses other drugs, or tell him to go out there and come back when things get bad enough? Perhaps the client has been involved with other counselors, one of whom said, "Okay, we're going to monitor your drinking and we're going to set up indicators of things that are out of control." When even one "authority" gives tacit approval of drinking, the cocaine addict will use this to try to persuade others to approve also.

Unawareness of Complete Drug Use Pattern

Usually when a cocaine addict says, "But you can't take away the alcohol and pot because they were never a problem," he has a poor perception of his actual drug consumption. What I have found is that their perception of alcohol and pot use predates their heavy cocaine use. Their model of how much is drunk or smoked may be one, two, or even five years old. It isn't current. One of the things you must do is capture the truth and drive it home.

First, I do a drug and alcohol history. A few days later I do a psycho-social history. Then I collapse the two together and say, "My, isn't this interesting. It looks like, as you escalated in your drug use, you also escalated in your psycho-social problems. And there also appears to be some escalation in the alcohol and pot use." This is an issue you will run into again and again.

Working toward *acceptance* of the *polydrug* problem should lead patients to the realization that they cannot use drugs of any kind.   Cocaine addiction has been devastating.   They owe money. They have lost almost everything they loved. They are in therapy, depressed, and extremely dysphoric, and yet there is a big piece of them that would like to use cocaine. They know that maybe they can't. But they remain unwilling to face the issues of alcohol and pot.

If a cocaine addict continues to use alcohol and pot, he will continue to use very poor judgment. And probably he will have a *relapse*. I have worked with clients on an *outpatient* basis, allowing them to define for themselves what out-of-control means in terms of pot and alcohol use. We have monitored drug use and I've kept them in treatment this way. When things start to go wrong, we begin working with the other addictions.

PSYCHIATRIC DISORDERS

Probably ten percent or more of those seeking treatment for cocaine dependence have psychiatric disorders. There is a relationship in the psychological literature suggesting that people who have certain psychological or psychiatric problems gravitate toward cocaine. I have mentioned that many drugs can be used to cope with problems. I don't know if you realize this, but the treatment on the street, which was the old treatment of choice in Europe for psychosis, was morphine. Morphine can knock someone right out of a psychotic episode. Heroin will do the same thing.

Sometimes a client doesn't fit your model of what a typical cocaine addict should look like. For example, I had a cocaine addict who was toxic and came in somewhat psychotic. He was having delusions and was in a paranoid state. He said, "I know that you people have planted a little radio in my molar, and that everyone in the waiting room can hear everything I am thinking."

This isn't a typical presentation of someone who is toxic and paranoid from cocaine. That is a typical presentation of schizophrenia. Schizophrenic is what this person was.

One of the things I ask is, "What were your subjective experiences when you first used cocaine? What was it like the first time?" They usually experience stimulation because cocaine is a central nervous system stimulant. Then, after about forty-five minutes to one hour, the person returns to his or her original state. There may be a slight *dysphoric rebound*. I've had several patients who ended up with depression problems tell me that they had a more pronounced rebound. This may be only a slight indicator, but it is something to be sensitive to.

Other psychiatric problems that may be encountered are bi-polar disorders, attention-deficiency disorders, *cyclothymic disorders,* and clinical depression. Of these, depression appears to be the most prevalent.

Depression

In the cocaine population you may find some pre-existing chronic depression. When you start to see someone who has these features, you will want to know about the family history and any depressive episodes that they may have had in the past. You will want to do a thorough history to document whether depressive episodes existed before the onset of cocaine usage.

The other phenomenon you will see is cocaine users fitting the model of bipolar illness—those who are *manic-depressive.* This condition must always be verified or ruled out, if suspected. This is to make sure that a psychiatric problem isn't going to become part of the problem once we begin treating the cocaine addiction. In cases where there is more pathology than just the addiction, we must treat the multiple conditions in a *parallel* fashion. If people find a drug that meets some of their needs, bio-chemical and psychological, the use of that drug is doubly entrenched.

Treating the addiction without treating the depression or other psychiatric problems is doomed to fail. As soon as you treat the cocaine problem they may become profoundly depressed. What are they going to think about? What type of *craving* are they going to have? I think when we consider these problems we begin to understand the bonds between psychiatric disorders and drug addiction.

INSTANT GRATIFICATION

Imagine that you are an adolescent or young adult. You've learned that in seconds you can feel better. Then I'd like you to imagine that one day someone said to you, "You really shouldn't use cocaine. You should find a softer, easier way of living. You should find a better, healthier way of life. Maybe you should try *Narcotics Anonymous (NA)* or *Cocaine Anonymous (CA)* or *Alcoholics Anonymous (AA)*. The next time you feel lonely, or isolated, or depressed, instead of picking up that freebase pipe that will make you feel better in six to eight seconds, why don't you just go to a meeting?"

Six seconds to instant gratification. The brain has learned that it can feel better quickly. Cocaine's expediency is a big obstacle to recovery.

Chapter 4

THE CRISIS

* Out-of-Balance Lives
* How Cocaine Dependents View Themselves
* Control Reversal
    - Aversive Conditioning
    - Contingency Contracting
    - A Positive Approach
* Motivational Crisis
    - Losses
    - Physical Problems
    - Psychological Problems
    - Keeping the Pain Level Up
* Life Stabilization Management
* Establishing the Concept of Addiction

John had reached a point in his cocaine addiction where he was chronically dysphoric. The only time he felt good or even normal was when he was freebasing.

John's family had left him weeks ago and he was on the verge of being fired. This didn't concern him as much as that he had used all of his family's savings in the last six months, owed nearly five thousand dollars to cocaine dealers and couldn't get cash for more of the drug.

In desperation, John accepted the offer of an acquaintance he had met in a local bar. This person, Mike, has asked John to sell him an ounce of cocaine. Mike had sixteen hundred dollars cash, the money necessary to score such an amount. John, using poor judgment due to his craving for cocaine, consented. He knew he could cut the cocaine and get an eight ball (one-eighth ounce of cocaine) for himself.

John met Mike in a predetermined spot—a grocery store parking lot at a shopping mall. While delivering the cocaine, an unmarked squad car sped to the scene. John had sold cocaine to an undercover police officer.

Only six months ago John was a respectable middle class plant maintenance worker. He had a lovely wife and two beautiful children. Now he had lost his job, family, and perhaps his freedom. But John was fortunate. As part of his sentencing, he was offered treatment and probation as an alternative to jail. The *bust* served as a motivator to force him to seek treatment.

OUT-OF-BALANCE LIVES

Even before a cocaine dependent experiences a *motivational crisis,* you begin seeing a life out-of-balance. Most of us, when we are feeling good and our lives are stable, perceive ourselves as having some control over our internal and external environments. When we feel in control our self-esteem is good, too. This isn't typical for the cocaine dependent.

For the cocaine dependent, a drug has provided the excitement. In using the drug, he has neglected the everyday details that help maintain home, family, self-respect, or job—the things we perceive as wonderful in our lives. A difficult challenge for treatment is to teach cocaine dependents how to maintain home, family, self-respect and job while still meeting needs for excitement and thrills. We must be sure to include this dimension in our treatment plan, along with working with the family. This is a good illustration of why it is so desirable to get the family involved in the treatment program.

HOW COCAINE DEPENDENTS VIEW THEMSELVES

Cocaine dependents don't see themselves as junkies. They see themselves as productive people. This is in direct contrast to many of the stereotypes of drug users. Although cocaine use is pervasive in lower socio-economic areas, the clients seen in private practice or clinics more often conform to this general profile: 29 year-old female or 30 year-old male; many earning $25,000 a year; spending $500-$700 per week on cocaine.

These people see themselves as still productive, capable of producing income and governing their lives. Even when they seek treatment, there is a part of them that still wants desperately to use cocaine. That paradox exists in all drug dependents who seek treatment, regardless of the substance of abuse. That paradox is extraordinarily strong in the cocaine addict—protected by control and power urges. The more power and control issues there are, the more difficult it is to motivate the cocaine addict to accept *inpatient* treatment. To surrender one's independence, even temporarily, is seen as a personal defeat.

CONTROL REVERSAL

The earliest recovery phase, "control reversal," begins when the *denial* of the drug problem is pierced and the painful realities of addiction start to break through. The cocaine dependent becomes intensely conscious that there is a problem. The escalation of environmental pressures—social, personal, legal and economic—is prerequisite to the personal growth stages of treatment.

While becoming dependent on cocaine, the person has developed an elaborate system of defense—especially denial and projections—a beautiful way of minimizing what is going on. As cocaine dependents they have developed a way of pigeon holing things. They keep one problem in this corner, another problem on the job in another corner, and some other nasty items tucked back somewhere else. Never shall they all meet.

The building environmental pressures, however, begin to break down some of the denial and the system starts to fail. We start to see a person who is literally sick. There is no longer any doubt that something is wrong. Yet the therapist, or anyone else trying to help, is still on the receiving end of all the defenses they have built up to avoid the painful reality of addiction.

An interesting part of this is the ambivalence. Cocaine use remains attractive even after massive losses, and even while in the process of admitting the problem and seeking help. Rarely do cocaine dependents come to a clinic and talk about psychosocial issues and inpatient care. All they may claim to be looking for is relief from the physical complaints. Outpatient remedies are often sought.

Aversive Conditioning

When I look at all the practices used by different people in different clinical settings to help the cocaine dependent regain control, there are some I am critical of. I see some attempts at reinventing the wheel, trying to do the same thing we tried to do with the alcoholic fifteen or twenty years ago. Even when these coercive control strategies work, they are contrary to the psychological principles of acceptance of the addiction, and more consistent with the *will power* model, long since proven unsuccessful.

I have read some of the accounts of *aversive conditioning* with intravenous heroin and cocaine addicts. They tell them little stories, like they just took a *"hot shot"* (battery acid, instead of cocaine). "You are starting to melt from the inside out and you're turning into a pile of crap. Your junkie friends don't want to have anything to do with you and throw you out in the street." You know, it's the old "barf therapy," aversive conditioning. I don't believe the approach is effective.

Contingency Contracting

A related technique, whose reports fill the literature on drug therapy, is *contingency contracting*. The greatest contingency contractor was Ben Franklin. Ben was involved in doing some of the early work on the frontier. Once he was building a fort, and the minister came up to him and said, "Ben, I just can't get people to come up and go through my services. What can I do?" Ben said, "No Problem." He suggested that they distribute rum at the end of each religious service. So from then on the church was packed. If you didn't go to church, you didn't get your portion of rum. In a way, that is a positive approach to conditioning; getting people to do something and then meeting one of their perceived needs. We don't give a cocaine dependent rum, but we can use other rewards.

Contingency contracting, as practiced in drug therapy, usually has an adverse consequence. You monitor a person's urine to determine if they have been using. If they have been using drugs, some undesirable but agreed to event, outlined in a preexisting contract, occurs. In one example, a C.P.A. agrees to write a letter to his accreditation board stating:

> *Dear Sir,*
>
> *I am a cocaine addict and my life is totally out of control. I urge you to revoke my license to practice as a C.P.A in this state.*

This letter is given to the therapist. He holds it over the client's head. If the client happens to relapse, the letter is sent to the certification board.

A Positive Approach

I believe that contingency contracts of this type should be used only as a last resort. What I prefer is a more positive approach to the modification of behaviors; positive instead of negative contingencies. I find that my clients respond well to goals and direction. So I try to turn the whole contracting process around. I begin by establishing simple goals, and reward their completion. I like that approach because it builds an ability to delay gratification. This is a skill that is underdeveloped in many cocaine dependent people.

I always try to understand the reward system of each cocaine dependent. For some it is money. For others it may be position or family. Find the rewards that act as reinforcers to the therapeutic process and you will be more successful in helping the cocaine dependent recover.

MOTIVATIONAL CRISIS

A reversal in control, similar to what I have described, occurs in just about any addiction. The alcoholic experiences a motivational crisis, but the cocaine dependent generally has more legal and financial complications to deal with.

Losses

The typical cocaine dependent has exhausted vast sums of money. And the loss of money is a motivational factor that will be a big part of what gets him into treatment. You can't do $150,000 worth of alcohol in six months, but you can easily do that much cocaine. There are people spending five thousand dollars or more per week on cocaine; some do an ounce of cocaine in a day. Freebasing? Sixteen hundred to two thousand dollars a day. At this rate available funds are exhausted fast. Credit is stretched to its limit.

Loss of family, friends and job is a powerful motivator, but even more destabilizing is involvement in illegal and immoral acts to support the cocaine addiction. These activities precipitate self-reexaminations that are agonizing. For both male and female, prostitution is often involved in supporting cocaine dependency. Whether it is overt or covert, prostitution causes intense feelings of guilt and shame. Being arrested, if you perceive yourself as a middle-class citizen, is devastating, too.

Physical Problems

Preoccupation with physical complaints is characteristic of the cocaine dependent's first attempts at seeking help. I repeatedly hear questions like, "I had a seizure once, will I have it again? That's all I want to know." Or, "I have a whole bunch of problems breathing through my nose because of snorting cocaine—and what I really want to know is, what is going to happen next?" You see a constellation of physical problems. Seizures are particularly scary and motivating. If they happened once they are likely to happen again, sometimes at lower doses and possibly even after the person has stopped using drugs.

Chronic fatigue, headaches, sore throats—all these physical symptoms are tied to abusing a central nervous system stimulant. To avoid these effects, other drugs are used. A user is freebasing; it's 2 A.M. He must get up at 6 A.M. to make a 7 A.M. job. He can't sleep without using a central nervous system depressant. If he uses a depressant he will wake up fatigued. These are some of the more common physical problems contributing to the motivational crisis of the cocaine dependent.

Psychological Problems

The continued use of most drugs leads to occasional feelings of depression and anxiety. We know from research literature on alcohol that a person who drinks in a bar becomes more depressed as he continues to drink through the evening.

Depression is often a result of changes in bio-chemistry brought on by drug use. People who use cocaine deplete the stimulating *neurotransmitters* in their brains—such as *dopamine*. (A characteristic of Parkinson's Disease is low levels of dopamine.) When people have low dopamine levels they typically feel depressed. They do not experience joy. The symptom is called *anhedonia*, from the word hedonism, meaning pursuit of joy.

Persons who have used cocaine excessively have depleted neurotransmitters in the brain. They feel depressed and remorseful about all the money they've spent. They may even have an agitated depression because the fire is still being stoked in there—but there isn't much dopamine left to lift the spirit. So they start feeling depressed, anxious, and irritable.

Paranoia is a phenomena seen in conjunction with the use of stimulants, that you don't see as often with depressant-type drug dependencies. With amphetamines, for example, you can get *amphetamine psychoses*—amphetamine types of paranoia. These tend to last longer than cocaine paranoias. From what I have seen, if there is no other overt psychiatric problem, paranoia stemming from excessive cocaine use will rapidly decrease along with decreases in the body's cocaine level.

The cocaine dependent's paranoia is usually "context appropriate." It is based on dangers inherent in the person's life, but exaggerated. If I fear being busted by the IRS or the Narcs, those are the people that I think are in my closet. Cocaine addicts always tell stories of sitting at home at two o'clock in the morning. "I hear a car go by and I know it must be the police. So I run to the window to look out. The whole night is a progression of going back and forth to the window, checking the cars that go by to see if it is the police out there, instead of a passerby." The mind goes crazy. It starts to play on those fears, exaggerating them. As soon as you take the drug away, the paranoia usually clears up. You may have occasional signs of it for a few days. Some people talk about having it for a few weeks.

You can use that paranoia in a treatment program. Low levels of paranoia can be a tool for you. If a client is afraid that someone at work is going to do something bad, talk about all the ways to guard against having that happen. You play with what each person gives you. "What can you do to keep that supervisor from getting on you? You can always let them know if you have to leave early. You can always take appropriate breaks; come back from lunch on time, show up in the morning on time." You can work with some of the paranoia as long as it does not interfere with that person's ability to do required daily activities.

Keeping the Pain Level Up

The motivational crisis is induced by pain. When the cocaine dependent person enters this important crossroad it is necessary to keep the pain level elevated. Don't tell them, "You are going to be okay." Don't tell them, "Just hang in there." I believe trying to find painless ways to change is an unproductive approach to drug addiction therapy. Pain is an important part of the recovery process. Even when a client comes in and says, "My life is worthless, my life is out of control," I look at them and say, "Yes you're right. And some areas may be even worse than you think they are." This sets the stage for keeping the pain level up. It may be the only motivational tool you have.

LIFE STABILIZATION MANAGEMENT

In Chapter Three I talked about finding the big picture by doing a "Columbo-type" technique. Besides an alcohol and drug history, I recommend doing a thorough psychosocial assessment and then merging the two, looking for problems and patterns. When we combine a psychosocial history of the client with his alcohol and drug history, a more revealing picture of the chemical dependency problem emerges than from either technique alone. Neither of these information gathering activities are just paperwork exercises. They both provide essential facts for planning a recovery program.

When I do a psychosocial assessment I don't like to bring up the results of the alcohol-drug assessment. I don't ask, "How much did you drink and how much did you drug when you were going through the first divorce?" These questions are guaranteed to trigger defensive reactions. Once a client is stabilized, I try to do an alcohol-drug assessment involving self-ratings in reaction to highly specific questions like: "When was your first use of cocaine? How much did you use in your early twenties and early thirties? I start building a chrono-logical picture of drug and alcohol use. Comparing this with the psychosocial history captures the chronology, the historical development of problems. By collapsing the two, I can start to break down some of the pigeon holing of different types of problems that is so common among cocaine dependents.

This is the big picture. When the therapist and the client together consider these facts, they start to see causal relationships between the use of cocaine and other drugs, and psychosocial problems with their job, family, and the law. I find it best to wait a few days between doing the drug-alcohol assessment and the psychosocial assessment. I usually do the psychosocial history as a self-assignment. I have them do it in their own room at night and then bring it in and talk about it.

I also do a life stabilization management process with a client who is in the crisis stage. It provides a foundation for all the therapy that is done later. It involves getting an accurate picture of the client's lifestyle and drugs of choice. Later, I talk with them about why people make the choices they do, and work toward stabilizing and maintaining their life.

Once the treatment program begins, I watch for patients who come in and say things like "Things just aren't the same as they used to be. I am just not feeling very good today." Maybe something has happened, a subjective experience of distress. They don't know what it is, so they look around and create a crisis. This helps the brain explain what the body is feeling.

One of the most interesting lessons I learned was while working with an alcoholic, about eight years ago. He came to me and said, "I just can't talk to you today because my son is smoking pot." Now, we hear that sometimes. Believing, I did a wonderful intervention on the family and got the kid into treatment. Dad relapsed.

The dad relapsed because I was so naive at the time that I did not turn that subjective distress back to him and talk to him about what was going on in his life. I "bought" what he told me hook, line and sinker, that the son was the problem. Actually, the son had been smoking pot for ten years. It was never an issue until then. The rule I learned is simple: Whenever you see a recovering person getting out of balance, especially the cocaine dependent, he will start to create excitement. *He will create a life crisis.*

ESTABLISHING THE CONCEPT OF ADDICTION

The cocaine dependent has two different people sitting on his shoulder. These represent conflicting feelings. One is saying, "Get the hell out of here." And then there is that strong side that says, "You're in the right place." A basic treatment challenge is to find the leverage you need to keep a person in treatment, when the weak side rears its ugly head and says, "Get the hell out of here because you know that would make you feel better."

My sense is that we must start to work with cocaine dependents during the motivational period, implanting the concept that they are ill. Even the way we give them valium should be consistent with this. I never say, " This pill will make you better." I say something like, "This pill will help you manage yourself better." The way you say things is critically important.

Beginning with the earliest treatment encounters with the cocaine dependent, a sensitive therapist or counselor searches for clues to "What is going on inside that person that will enable him to see himself as chemically dependent, and to help him become comfortable with that idea?"   At this time, you probably can only hope to establish an addiction concept for cocaine. Consideration of other drugs used, the alcohol and the pot, will occur later. So, right from the start, getting the concept of addiction implanted and trying to get the cocaine dependent into the appropriate level of care is essential in creating a foundation for recovery.

Chapter 5

EARLY TREATMENT ENCOUNTERS

* Indicators of Toxicity
    - Overdose: Mild to Moderate Symptoms
    - Cocaine Psychosis
    - Hyperpyrexia
* Detoxification
    - Fighting
    - Withdrawal Symptoms
    - Medications for Withdrawal
    - Need for Patient Monitoring
    - Self-Medication
    - Outpatient Treatment
* Intake
    - Worst Case Scenario Building
    - Using the Appeal of Specialness
    - The Special Unit Advantage
    - The Identification Process
    - Illustrating the Intake Process
* The Outpatient Option
    - Old Friends Can Bring You Down
    - How to Relate to Drug-Using Friends
* The SIPIO Option

Let's consider someone who is freebasing one thousand dollars worth of cocaine per week. Our primary concern now is detoxification and dealing with the behavioral correlates of toxicity and withdrawal. Detoxification is usually the first requirement in cocaine dependency treatment. Some cocaine users require detoxification but don't want to enter inpatient treatment because they see it as too restrictive. They may also be poor candidates for, or resist continuing, outpatient treatment. One thing is almost certain: *a one-shot outpatient visit doesn't work* for people who are compromised by chronic cocaine addiction. Intake into a carefully structured treatment program should follow the motivational crisis.

INDICATORS OF TOXICITY

A prime indicator of toxicity is agitation. The person just cannot stay still. Instead of the psychomotor retardation characteristic of alcoholic intoxication, cocaine toxics are "all over the place." They show some grandiosity, elation, and they tend to talk a lot. They are distractible. Their auditory acuity appears heightened. They hear sounds that other people do not hear and may react to them with fear and paranoia. I described this hypervigilance as a "Ping Pong match" phenomena. Hypervigilance is often followed by paranoia that, as we have said, is context-apropriate.

Overdose: Mild to Moderate Symptoms

Mild to moderate symptoms of cocaine overdoses are often ignored by the person using cocaine. They reach a point, after snorting, freebasing or injecting for a considerable period of time, where almost reverse effects from the cocaine appear. I have heard addicts say, "I get this strange, funny feeling at times, this general feeling of malaise. Sometimes I can just keep snorting or freebasing and I can work my way through it." The other thing described is profuse perspiration. I saw a fellow perspire so profusely that you could watch the sweat bead up on his toes and fingers. They will just drip and run sweat. This is not always from a massive overdose, but from a moderate overdose.

I remember sitting in an airport in 1971 and breaking out in a sweat. In less than five minutes the sweat was dripping off me.

I sneaked off to the bathroom every fifteen minutes while waiting for the plane. I reached a point where I had moderate symptoms of cocaine overdose. I remember watching all the people watching me. I tried to explain to them that I had the flu.

Clients should be asked about reverse effects and sweating because they are mild symptoms of overdose. It is not the full-blown toxic episode. You see more profound types of problems with cocaine when you get into the higher dose levels — especially with freebasers and I.V.-users. High-dose users sometimes report *pseudo-hallucinations* such as "*snow lights*," flicks of white or silver light in the peripheral vision field.

Cocaine Psychosis

In *cocaine psychosis,* many people will *hallucinate.* As long as you are in control of them this isn't a problem. There are many variations of the bizarre. I can remember talking to a relative who wasn't there. Another time, I remember a friend of mine reporting the actual conversation he had with another friend. That friend was one hundred miles away, but the conversation was so vivid and clear, it was real.

Another symptom of cocaine psychosis is seeing "*cocaine bugs.*" The bugs may appear to be anywhere in the room, even on the person's skin. One client brought a piece of his own flesh in a vial, just so he could convince a medical doctor that there actually were cocaine bugs under his skin. This phenomenon is similar to *delirium tremens (D.T.s)* seen in the withdrawing alcoholic.

Hyperpyrexia

There are some other toxic complications worth mentioning. A person who is using too much cocaine can die because of elevated body temperature. The body temperature can reach 107 or 108 degrees and stay there. This condition is called *hyperpyrexia* and it is one way that people die from cocaine overdose. Treatment for hyperpyrexia involves providing life support systems and body cooling. *Thorazine* is sometimes used to block some of the heat build up. But, if a person is prone to seizure, thorazine can be dangerous because it lowers the seizure threshold. A person taking thorazine can enter into "*status epilepticus,*" repeated grand mal seizures. When you start to get into status epilepticus, you don't get enough oxygen into your brain. Severe brain damage can result.

DETOXIFICATION

Detoxification involves withdrawal from the intoxicating substances. Cocaine detoxification requires careful, professional management, expecially when there is fear of central nervous system-depressant withdrawal. Usually the toxicity subsides on its own with time. However, the client should be in a supervised setting where competent medical care is immediately available. Chemical restraints may be required to treat the patient humanely and prevent self-inflicted injuries.

Fighting

The *Diagnostic and Statistical Manual* of the American Psychiatric Association (DSM-III) tends to emphasize the belligerency and aggression associated with intoxication from any drug. From what I've observed, a drug in and of itself doesn't directly cause anything except impaired judgment. Sometimes the impaired judgment may lead to fighting. Interference with social functioning is, of course, associated with intoxication and this is described in detail in the APA's *Diagnostic and Statistical Manual.*

Withdrawal Symptoms

I believe that cocaine is a physically addictive substance, and that withdrawal produces a readily observable set of behaviors. Withdrawal from cocaine looks almost, at times, like people getting a little stuporous from taking too many central nervous system depressants. It is a phenomenon of the sympathetic nervous system. Typically, we see considerable confusion and, initially, dysphoria. Then, after twenty-four to forty-eight hours, you start to see profound depression, often accompanied by headaches, irritability and sleep disturbances.

Medications for Withdrawal

What medications are given to ease cocaine withdrawal? There is no highly effective drug that I've seen given for cocaine withdrawal. The symptoms of withdrawal are what is actually treated. For example, if the person has an agitated depression with difficulty sleeping, valium may be prescribed by the attending physician. The medications I have seen used most are the *benzodiazepines,* to deal with the discomfort of early withdrawal.

Diagnosing withdrawal from the cocaine addiction has sometimes been complicated by the presence of a central nervous system depressant, such as alcohol or valium, or any tranquilizing or sleep medications. A person who is already on high doses of valium must be slowly weaned from that.

During withdrawal, *tricyclic anti-depressants* are used also. Theoretically, they increase the level of dopamine in the brain. They ease the depression and drug craving that may be a by-product of some of a person's nasty feelings. There are reports that excessive sleeping during withdrawal (*hypersomnia* or lethargy) is corrected by trycyclic anti-depressants. *Lithium* has been researched, too. Others have tried the use of *tyrosine* and *tryptophan,* naturally occurring amino acids. They are the precursors of stimulatory neuro-transmitters (dopamine, for example), and some of the stimulatory neuro-transmitters (*serotonin, norepinephrine*) depleted during cocaine use.

Need for Patient Monitoring

My real concern (especially if considerable anguish is involved and there is any past history of self-destructive behavior) is that the person withdrawing from cocaine be monitored closely. The potential for self-destructive behavior is there. I think we should always remain alert to this possibility.

Self-Medication

People have a history of medicating themselves. Earlier I mentioned the use of heroin and opiates to treat cocaine psychosis and other psychoses. In working with cocaine dependent clients, you will see the "street cure" for this. Pot, alcohol, valium or any of the opiates, especially heroin, help them deal with some of the side effects of cocaine toxicity. As the cocaine starts to clear from the blood you will see the toxicity clear up. About the only time you must intervene is if a person completely loses contact with reality. If you look into their eyes, and there's "no one home," or there's "someone else at the wheel," they are having a psychotic episode. Episodes of this depth mandate a structured, inpatient clinical environment.

Outpatient Treatment

In an area such as San Francisco, where there are few treatment beds, cocaine psychosis is sometimes treated on an outpatient basis. They often administer *haldol* several times a day, and bring addicts in for counseling—just for reality grounding. Although you will see psychotic behaviors, they are usually transient. Many patients will tell me that they love to reach a point where they start to hallucinate. They enjoy that aspect. It doesn't trouble them.

INTAKE

Let's assume that the client has gone through a toxic episode. Now we're concerned with introducing him to the treatment center, while trying to keep him from turning away from a recovery program. In my experience, many clients undergoing detoxification withdraw from treatment within the first three days. This is unfortunate because detoxification must be repeated later. Our first priority is to prevent this person from leaving the treatment program during the first two or three days they are there. I have found that any isolation of the client tends to promote leaving the treatment program.

It is never easy to get the cocaine addict to recognize the need for inpatient treatment. You are dealing with the control needs of the individual. If this is the case, there's no way to help other than keeping the pain level up, trying to keep the family from enabling them, establishing a concept of addiction, and starting to move toward the goal of in-depth acceptance.

Having the right person available at intake can make the difference between an addict starting a successful recovery program, or backing away. In directing clinical programs I have always made it a policy to identify the staff who are most effective at assessment-intake. You must have an excellent counselor at the assessment-intake interface because it demands considerable sensitivity and inter-personal skill.

Worst Case Scenario Building

Something I have found to cause problems is when people in pain are allowed to isolate themselves, they make the worst case out of everything. If you are waiting for your boy friend or girl friend, and he or she is thirty minutes late, what do you tend to do if you are sitting there by yourself? You play worst case. You build a worse case out of everything. Similarly, strong impulses to leave treatment can be a direct result of the patient's having been left alone to build worst cases.

If you have a cocaine addict you're bringing through the intake process, and you say, "Go sit in room 167 and the nurse will be in to take care of you," it may take fifteen to twenty minutes for the nurse to get there. By that time, you may have someone profoundly emotional and scared, who has built himself to a point where he's ready to walk out of the treatment program. The best way to work with addicts on an inpatient basis is by direct transfer of care, from the direct supervision of one staff member to another.

Using The Appeal of Specialness

To the cocaine dependent the appeal of specialness is incredible. In truth, they are chemically addicted, just like so many others. Knowing this, you can sometimes come up with ways to turn their exaggerated sense of specialness into something positive for recovery. If the sense of specialness is all the client will give me to work with, I use it however I can to help him.

Sometimes you can make leading comments that appeal to that specialness. I know that when I start to work with someone, I have two tasks. One task is to create some structure in his life. The second is to provide some initiative. The structure is the treatment program, but how do you draw that person in and keep him coming back?

I have used this approach successfully: The person with a cocaine problem calls on the phone to ask about treatment. I'll say, "Yes, the person who referred you called me and told me about you. They said you were very special, and that you move quite quickly. I only take people who move quickly." If you want to see a glow on someone's face, watch the cocaine addict when you say this. They want to be perceived as special.

I am reminded of a very beautiful, twenty-eight year old woman. I was sitting there talking to her. She had been on the unit about twelve hours and was going through the confusion and dysphoria that accompanies cocaine withdrawl. She had a three thousand dollar a week habit and had been prostituting herself from drug dealer to drug dealer to support her habit. She was sitting there, looking at me with her mascara running, weeping, and bent over. A fifty year old alcoholic walks through the door and this lady pulls herself up, and stands up and says, "I do three thousand dollars of cocaine a week. What do you do?" This is self-perception of specialness.

The Special Unit Advantage

If you have a special cocaine treatment unit available, it goes a long way toward selling the cocaine dependent on inpatient treatment. A unit of this type conveys an image of uniqueness. A special unit to meet the needs of the cocaine dependent has proven to be economically feasible in larger hospitals or multiple treatment facilities. They are quickly filled and have waiting lists. We have two with waiting lists in Chicago at the time of this writing.

The Identification Process

If you have clients coming in, seeing themselves as special—but not belonging—one of the things to do is to "get them hooked into" other cocaine people. This way they can know "We are not alone. We're not the only people who have this problem." You start the process of identification.

In an inpatient environment there is structure. We have *milieus, self-help* meetings, structured time. We can organize this administratively, but initiative is the part we must create in our interaction with the clients. Providing structure and taking the initiative means dealing with the specialness, getting them involved, and bringing them to see themselves as part of the unit, not as an extra cog. Once they begin to see this happen, as they start to work in the milieu, in their meetings and self-help groups, they will start to develop a sense of hope. They will see people who are like them, with the same problems, doing better. If we start working with the initiative, dealing with the specialness, going ahead and playing with that narcissistic child inside, we will have better luck at "keeping them in the ball game."

Take the patients into the day room, into the milieu, and introduce them to at least two or three other cocaine or polydrug addicted persons. Get them to start telling *drug-a-logues.* That is their common denominator at this time. Hope arises from their knowing their problem is not unique, and that others share their problems and aspirations for recovery.

Illustrating the Intake Process

If I was the intake person, the first thing I would do is work with the concept of addiction. I would try to keep the pain level up, but I would take the patient and directly introduce him to the nurse who would be doing the physical nursing assessment. I think that is crucial, a good transfer of care. The nurse does her assessment, then introduces the patient to the technician or a counselor-assistant who can do the belonging search.

Next, I would introduce the primary counselor, so we can start to lay the ground work and get this person involved. I would say to the cocaine dependent, "There is a part of you that wants to leave, isn't there?" (And you know this is a big part of him, at this early stage.) "There is also a part of you that brought you in here, and knows what is best for you. Is that not so? I want to congratulate you on that strong side of you, because only ten to fifteen percent of the cocaine dependents have the guts to come in and face their problem." Appeal to that specialness. Say, "You are special. You are one of the few people who has the guts to come and do what you are doing. When that ugly part of you rears that ugly head, I want you to contract to sit down and talk to me before making any decisions."

THE OUTPATIENT OPTION

Do we have any criteria to judge when a person should enter inpatient vs. outpatient treatment? What about the possibility of outpatient treatment for someone who has lost control of his behavior through dependency, but still has a healthy family? The cocaine dependent says he is willing to enter Alcoholics Anonymous and Cocaine Anonymous, and is willing to work through weekly outpatient counseling. Is he doomed to fail? Possibly.

If you look at outpatient treatment, there are few indicators showing that outpatient treatment once a week with cocaine addicts is successful, even if the family is intact and supportive. The prognosis is even worse if there are any medical or psychiatric complications. A person displaying a psychotic episode generally needs inpatient stabilization. If he is having seizures, he also requires inpatient services. When he is in an environment that is not healthy enough to support a recovery program, you are setting him up for failure if you put him right back in that old environment. All the *anchors* and cues remain there.

Old Friends Can Bring You Down

There is usually no healthy subset of friends for the early recovering cocaine dependent in an outpatient program. The people they will associate with are the same as before they entered treatment. A problem you run into if you put a person back into an unhealthy subset is that these friends are likely to have a vested interest in undermining the person's recovery program. Friends of the recovering cocaine dependent too often use this logic: "I run with you all the time and you and I don't have a problem. All of a sudden you say to yourself, 'I have a problem,' and go into treatment. What does that say about me? I have to do some self-evaluation. What am I going to do the next time you come around? If you are doing well, and we used to run together, and now you say that you have a problem, I'm going to try to pull you down to my level. Then neither of us has a problem. When I have to introspect myself and evaluate myself based on you, and you are doing well, that makes me feel bad."

How to Relate to Drug-Using Friends

Practicing how to relate to drug-using friends must be part of a treatment program. I often do this by surprise. I will have a person sit there and I'll just get up in his face and say, "You know I am a friend of yours. You know I have been with you for fifteen years and we have drugged for a long time. Who the hell are those people in the treatment center anyway? They have only known you for ten, fifteen, twenty days. Tell me about those pussies. Come on, we've been out on the street a long time. Come on, let's do a couple of lines." Verbally, he has no response because he's distraught by emotion. The intellect "goes right down the tubes." He can sit there and tell you, "What I would like to do is tell these people that if I'm really their friend they'd accept my addiction and support me." But you better get in his face and let him practice saying it. He must be comfortable with those statements—or in a real confrontation he will lose his good intentions. I am very careful about that, especially when clients come from an environment where they have to go back and be around people who are their *running set*.

What I think is needed is to give clients a progressive model of their cocaine dependence so that they can see themselves on the continuum. Make it a process, and not an event. In arranging outpatient treatment, develop a contract with the client that states that if the outpatient approach fails he will enter inpatient treatment. Define what failure means for the individual. "What does it mean for you to be out of control? What must happen for you to be able to see yourself as out of control?" The client may say that he can't get up and go to work anymore, or "I don't have money to pay the bills." *Clients must start to establish some way that, when they relapse on an outpatient basis, they can start to see themselves as part of a progressive model of addiction.*

I have had good results with a large number of snorters, and a few freebasers and injectors, seeing them two to three times a week for the first two to three months, on an outpatient basis. I have done that with people who have had no history of attempted suicide and who have no history of repeated failure on an outpatient basis. They should have some family support, although the family may be in denial or shock, experiencing some difficulty. There should be a willingness to become involved in Alcoholics Anonymous and Cocaine or Narcotics Anonymous, and no more than mild to moderate impairment in thought and emotional processes. If someone is grossly impaired in thinking and feeling, you cannot work with that person in an outpatient environment.

THE SIPIO OPTION
(Shortened Inpatient/Intensive Outpatient)

We should be aware that motivation is likely to be external in an inpatient treatment program. Also, clients will experience difficulties integrating with the inpatient environment. For these reasons alone, intensive outpatient programming is an attractive concept. I recommend that an effective alternative would combine the best of inpatient and outpatient approaches.

Begin the treatment program with a shortened inpatient stay, seven to fourteen days. During this inpatient period, undertake detoxification and assess the client for self-destructive behavior. You assess the environment and the family, stabilize the person, and begin some self-help work. Then it may be possible to put him into a more intensive outpatient environment, followed by basic counseling. This approach makes sense and may be the most cost-effective.

We have already begun to see shortened inpatient stays. This will become more prevalent as drug dependency treatment becomes a greater financial burden in the "private pay sector." It is on the way. In working with General Motors, I have seen their length of stay already fall two or three days. In the last year we have started to see more people exposed to intensive outpatient programming, but the programming must involve the family. It also must be aided by self-help, or generally it will not work.

Chapter 6

ACCEPTANCE IN DEPTH

* Working With Acceptance Issues
  -Powerlessness
  -Pain and Acceptance
* Discovering a Higher Power
* Resistance to Powerlessness
  -Will Power or Acceptance?
  -The Pull of Self-Defeating Behaviors
  -Testing Yourself or "Doing It the Hard Way"
* The Power of the *Milieu*
  -The Role of Anonymous Organizations
* Why Confrontation Doesn't Work
* Using the Self-Study Approach
  -Significant Memories
* The Two D's: Discipline and Dedication

WORKING WITH ACCEPTANCE ISSUES

A recovery program is demanding. What it boils down to is that we ask people to change everything, and to do it quickly. When we make this type of demand, and psychological defense systems remain active, problems will certainly follow. People begin looking around, not seeing themselves as ill with cocaine addiction. They start looking for excuses and external reasons for why they're who and where they are. If this happens, can we expect them to follow through on all our beautiful treatment plans?   No. The key to recovery is accepting that a problem exists and moving on from there.

Powerlessness

Let's look at what is probably the toughest part of the acceptance issue for the cocaine addict. People have a generalized notion of will power or impulse control. Our task as counselors is to help translate these generalized ideas into highly internalized concepts with personal meaning. In other words, we try to get the cocaine dependent to admit powerlessness over the chemical and be willing to ask for help. This is the foremost challenge of treating cocaine dependence. If achieved, the other parts of the program will fall into place. Without it, there is no consistent program. If a person accepts the reality of cocaine dependency, then we can start to work with changes in behaviors and attitudes. They will be open to change, and their energy will go into making those changes instead of defending the status quo.

Pain and Acceptance

Pain is a great motivator of acceptance. It is a direct, personal experience that you can't evade. You can't talk you're way out of it. The recovering cocaine addict's pain is rarely physical. It's a psychological pain emerging from a heightened awareness of the realities of damaged or destroyed family, social, occupational, legal, and economic status.

A counselor's role is to insure that these realities retain their high profile in the thinking and feeling of the early recovering cocaine addict. Harry Tiebout, in the early AA literature, said it this way: "When the unconscious forces of defiance and grandiosity actually cease to function effectively, the individual is wide open to reality. He can listen and learn without conflict and fighting back." I have found that when the pain level drops there is a strong tendency for the door to close—the door inward to feelings and consciousness, and the door outward toward healthier, adaptive patterns.

DISCOVERING A HIGHER POWER

To me, the whole key in treating any chemical dependency is working with this acceptance step. It isn't a concrete step, one that we can indisputably prove we're working on. I think that it is best represented as a major internal readjustment. We talk about it in terms of a higher power or good modeling. We talk about it in terms of involving a curative factor called "hope." We can look at it in several different ways. Fundamentally, however, it is a conversion process outside the direct control of client or counselor. We can only create the conditions that maximize the likelihood for acceptance to occur.

I am still amazed to see people suddenly become comfortable with being addicted. I find that this is a struggle for any chemically dependent person although the concepts are similar. What is acceptance and what does it mean when someone can "*let go and let God?*"

In early AA literature, in letters between Bill W. and Carl Yung, Carl talks about the alcoholic and says, "No matter what I did, nothing worked." He said that, then "something happened"—at which point the person had a conversion reaction or a spiritual conversion—and he became comfortable with his addiction. He was able to maintain a productive lifestyle without returning to drink.

RESISTANCE TO POWERLESSNESS

Consider *adult children* of alcoholics. They feel that their lives are out of control anyway, and they have no problem with the first step. "What do you mean powerless? I'm hopeless." The cocaine addict has just the opposite orientation. They have extreme difficulty *letting* something happen. To them, the concept of being involved in *making* something happen makes more sense.

Again we are involved with the issues of power and control. Cocaine addicts resist asking for help. They are accustomed to being in control and this behavior pattern diametrically opposes the first step: *admitting to powerlessness and the unman-ageability of life.*

Will Power or Acceptance?

I am interested in both non-verbal and verbal messages. There are two messages usually imparted. In terms of acceptance, I often look at the difference between "willing something to happen" and "becoming willing for something to happen." Using the will power model, a person will say to you, "I should be able to deal with this problem. I can handle what is going on in my life." I can, should, could, ought—all these are will power words. When a person starts to say these to you, it's a subtle indicator that he's working a different model from the one that usually works.

To create conditions conducive to developing acceptance, the counselor engages a person's mind in an awareness building process. I think about myself. "When does a person become comfortable with the personal awareness of cocaine addiction?" If you are a recovering person, what happened to you? Did you bang your head against the wall? Did you try to do it your way? You may have been one of the patients who, after three days, ran out and said, "I know exactly what to do now. I make three meetings a week and talk to my wife on Saturday nights. And it's all going to work out. I know exactly what to do now, and know how to control it." That is a flight into hell—a will power model, and nothing more. If you want to be miserable, try to treat chemical dependency with will power. It is very dangerous and leads to relapse.

The Pull of Self-Defeating Behaviors

If a person is functioning on will power alone, merely putting him in a stressful situation will cause the same old self-defeating thoughts and behaviors to return. You have a person who intellectually says, "Yes, I need to stay away from this stuff." But his emotions will override his intellect. And he is going to make some poor judgments. People who operate on a will power model test their abstinence more than those who accept powerlessness. If you think about it, the implication is:

"If I have will power I should be able to test this doggone thing and make it work."

Testing Yourself or "Doing it the Hard Way"

People "running on will power" put themselves around cocaine. They will go right out of the treatment center to a party where they know cocaine will be available. They will become overwhelmed. They will try to do everything the hard way. I often see this self-defeating pattern—attempting recovery the hard way—bargaining away everything helpful.

One of the things you will also find is that if you have a patient who is a perfectionist, is self-critical and has the "self talk" pattern—that everything I do I must work hard for, or it isn't good—he will probably want to test his abstinence. By putting himself in a position where cocaine is available, he is trying to recover the hard way. It's like the alcoholic who wants to go back into the bar and have ginger ale, because he wants to be with friends.

THE POWER OF THE *MILIEU*

What happens in the acceptance phase isn't totally between the therapist and the patient. It begins within the patient but requires peer interactions to develop. Patient-to-patient dialogue is crucial to the process. Acceptance is promoted when one patient is doing well and is modeling something that the other patient would like to have: stability in life.

Part of developing acceptance is becoming involved with winners. Counselors should try to expose the early recovering cocaine addict to other chemically dependent people who have struggled and dealt with the will power model. You can often structure a group so there is a person in it who is like your client, but who has worked through acceptance. You let them work together and see if growth occurs through modeling.

The Role of Anonymous Organizations

There are some organizational resources available to both inpatient and outpatient clients that foster acceptance. We have two major organizations for recovering cocaine dependents: Cocaine Anonymous and Narcotics Anonymous.

The newer one, Cocaine Anonymous, may require a cautious approach. My fear about Cocaine Anonymous is that at times people go into a Cocaine Anonymous group where the greatest amount of abstinence represented in the group is only six to nine months. There are no "old timers." The only resources that these novice abstainers may have are the old "drug-a-logues" and, "How I used to freebase." There isn't much abstinence value to these. In fact, they may create pressures for relapse, called "cravings."

Sometimes clients will call me from Cocaine Anonymous meetings and say, "What the hell are you doing to me? I got so hungry there, I had to leave." So, whenever possible, I encourage clients to become involved in Alcoholics Anonymous. It is an established organization with a varied cross-section of members. If there is any alcohol involved in the cocaine dependent's profile, and some willingness to give it up, AA is the modality I always use.   However, many AA members do not accept primary cocaine addicts. It is the therapist's job to initially place the patient in the right self-help group.

WHY CONFRONTATION DOESN'T WORK

Confronting a person's lack of acceptance isn't helpful. It doesn't work because it creates an "us against them" atmosphere. I share this idea with you because there is a part of every patient that hates the counselor or therapist.   Think about it. This person must come to the counselor because some part of his life is out of control. I have yet to meet anyone who likes to be out of control. What he is coming to you and saying is, "My life is out of control and therefore I need to come to you for help. I am glad you are there, but I am angry that I have to do this to begin with."   A successful counselor remains sensitive to the client's need to accept his drug dependency, recovery process and the counselor's persona. Hard confrontation undermines the acceptance of the counselor by the cocaine addict.

USING THE SELF-STUDY APPROACH

The initial task is to start to work with the acceptance issue and try to make some sense out of it. What may be helpful is returning to the AA literature. Unfortunately, there is still no established body of self-help material that deals specifically with cocaine dependency and recovery problems. There's a Narcotics Anonymous book out, but no Cocaine Anonymous book.

By carefully assigning readings about addiction, and observing client reactions to them, the therapist gains useful information. The things that jump out at us when we read do so because they are personally significant, meaningful or important. Why do we retain certain early memories? Because they are significant to us; they mean something to us. If we can get people to be unencumbered by their defense systems, then we can use some of Tiebout's work as a projective type of tool.

The Tiebout papers are pamphlets that cost about three dollars and fifty cents each. One of them talks about ego factors in early recovery. Another, which I use, is called *Surrender vs. Compliance.* I give it to the patient as a self-study assignment. But the way I frame the assignment is unconventional. I don't say, "Read this and tell me what parts apply to you; underline those and we will talk about it later." I put a different frame around it by saying, "Read this and, whatever interests you, just underline it and bring it in the next time you come. And bring my book back, Okay? Just underline whatever interests you."

What's the difference between telling the client to underline the parts that apply to him, and underline the parts that interest him? The latter frame does not trigger a defense strategy nearly as much as the former. That is important because what I want Tiebout's work to be is a projective test;

in other words, a reverse ink blot test. Things will jump out of that pamphlet at the individual for a reason: because they are significant.

Significant Memories

What will come in is little bits of underlined material that you can start to talk about. This is an opportunity to translate some of the generalized notions into the powerlessness concept. You tie the material they underline into the first step of Cocaine Anonymous or Alcoholics Anonymous, and start to talk in depth about issues such as a Higher Power and the willingness to ask for help.

THE TWO D's: DISCIPLINE AND DEDICATION

The foundation we build from day one of treatment, along with the daily personal program, are essential to recovery. Both are indispensable. If the foundation is lacking, or if someone is not working a healthy program, nothing that we do as therapists will work right. This person will slide and fall right in front of us. When we start to look at any recovery program, we always get down to discipline and dedication. There is no magic to recovery. It's doing all the little things, daily, that allows one to survive. Recovery is like running down an up-escalator. If you stand still you are losing ground.

Chapter 7

HELPING STRATEGIES

* An Educational Model for Cocaine
* The Alcohol and Marijuana Complication
    -A Case Study of Continued Alcohol
        and Pot Use
    --The Written Contract
    --Avoiding the Error of Multiple
        Abuse Models
    -The Odds of Maintaining Control
    -Group Reactions Reinforce
    -The Abstinence Dilemma
* Euphoric Recall
    -Triggers to Altered Consciousness
    -Reverse Rituals
    -Disassociating
* Finding Alternative Rewards
* Using Mental Imagery Effectively
* Nicotine, Coffee and Diet Pills
* Desensitizing to Cocaine Aroma
* When Cocaine is Part of a Relationship
    -Expanding Dimensions of Sexuality
    -Dealing With Guilt and Shame

Let's assume that a cocaine dependent is working on acceptance and has been through a motivational crisis. He is attending AA, NA or CA meetings, the family is in treatment, and progress is being shown in what we term early recovery. From here we start to work with some of the early treatment issues, planning the treatment approach based on the client's strengths.

I want to warn you that, once the client has reached this point, a common mistake is to say, "You're ready. Now go out and do." I'm not sure that we always tell people to "go out and do" based on their strengths. How to handle high risk situations may not yet have been dealt with in treatment. Often, at this stage, the client isn't aware of the cues and anchors of relapse. You have a person who walks back into their former environment—without a repertoire of alternative behaviors to help them deal with some of the issues of their addiction. Pushing the limits of these weaknesses in a treatment plan is a formula for failure. What we must do at this stage is implement an educational model that speaks directly to the cocaine dependent's unique problems.

AN EDUCATIONAL MODEL FOR COCAINE

How adequate for cocaine recovery is the educational model that prevails in most treatment centers originally established to treat alcoholics? Today, many alcohol treatment centers are making a transition into chemical dependency, but their educational model is still a chronic alcohol model. Like any job involving much training and experience, professionals in the alcohol treatment field don't change easily.

If you adhere to a middle-to-chronic alcohol model, you risk reinforcing the idea that the cocaine dependent does not belong in the treatment setting. A cocaine user doesn't see himself in the context of typical alcoholic problems. They have no liver damage. They have little end organ pathology. Cocaine addiction is a different dynamic and a different progression. This dilemma stems from a lack of specialized cocaine treatment facilities, and the resulting tendency to try to make the cocaine dependent, a square peg, fit into an alcohol treatment program, a round hole.

The other problems that alcohol treatment units have in serving cocaine dependents is that all their lectures are *Father Martin's Chalk Talks*. It is a wonderful movie and I love it. But it isn't meaningful and relevant to the cocaine dependent. You also have, "Let's talk about the progression of alcohol; let's talk about alcoholism, sexuality and recovery. Let's talk about alcoholism and...," because most staff members are recovering alcoholics and the program was developed on the basis of Alcoholics Anonymous.

Sex is a problem area that also must be dealt with in any educational model because cocaine is a profound aphrodisiac. You have acceptance problems when the cocaine addict escalates the use of alcohol and pot. Some of the return to work issues are different.   You rarely find alcoholics who owe twenty-five hundred dollars to people on the job.   And an educational model must address the internal and external cues and achors that are involved in relapse, things to watch out for, and how to change the pattern.

There's pressure to move to an addiction model because the hospital administrator perceives a need and a growing market for this service. However, to provide an effective treatment program for cocaine dependents, we must reexamine the whole education and self-help process. Alcohol treatment centers are doing a great job bringing in Narcotics Anonymous, but their educational models often need revising.

THE ALCOHOL AND MARIJUANA COMPLICATION

Generally, the use of a depressant drug predated the use of cocaine. When the cocaine became out of control, so did the use of marijuana and alcohol. I think that part of the technique is working with the issue of going back, and looking at the escalation of the alcohol and marijuana problems. What would you do with a person who came in to see you, who had been snorting cocaine—up to three to four hundred dollars per week?   You decide to treat them on an outpatient basis. They take the position, "Okay, I'm going to try to give up the cocaine, but don't talk to me about giving up the alcohol, and pot." How do you deal with that? What do you do?

You have two choices, two extreme choices. You say, "Okay, let's work on the cocaine problem and let's define what 'out of control' means for you, in regard to the alcohol and pot." Or you say, "I'm unwilling to work with you because I only work with people who believe in total abstinence." The second way, you lose them from any treatment. With the first option, you keep them in treatment and try to motivate them to take a closer look at their alcohol and pot use. One method of assessing control is asking them to prove their control by refraining from use for three to six months.

A Case Study of Continued Alcohol and Pot Use

As an example, I had a male client who was about twenty-nine years old. He was an aspiring drummer, very macho, and very handsome. What I tried to do was find out what in his life was valuable to him. This person had used cocaine for two years—all intranasal use. Things were going well for him until his marriage started to deteriorate. He didn't like some of the things that were going on in his life. His money flow had gotten bad and that had angered his wife. She threatened to leave and he came into treatment.

He came in and said, "Okay, now I want to work on an out-patient basis." I said, "I am willing, for the first two to three weeks, to see you three times a week. Then we will meet once a week for the next six months." I allowed him to go ahead and continue to drink and to smoke. I did it for this reason: my sense was that if I kept him in treatment, at least I had him in a place where I could monitor him. He had no problem saying cocaine was the only thing that he had ever lost control over. He was a very controlling gentleman. He was able to work with the cocaine very nicely.

I also treated him and his wife in couples counseling. I found that he used cocaine one time. It was a one shot instance about six weeks into his recovery. He convinced himself that he was just chasing an illusion and became a little bit discouraged. He called me up and we talked about it. In some ways it may have been a therapeutic relapse. He learned something from it. In the last seven or eight months he used no cocaine at all. But during the last two months his alcohol use escalated.

The Written Contract

I talked with him about a progressive model of alcohol use and the succession of events that happens to a person. We tied it into some similar phenomena with his cocaine addiction. And we developed a written contract which I linked to daily logs he kept of his activities. His contract stated that he was going to run three or four times a week, make so many meetings, practice drums six times a week, weigh every day, and bring the daily records in every time he came to see me. He could have lied to me—some people can do that with ease. This person, for a while, had no problem at all. He had a couple of beers, a glass of wine in the evening.

Then the alcohol started to progress. He was never "into" pot. I think that in the whole nine months he only smoked a couple of joints. Soon this man, who ran every day and practiced drums, began to skip both. He started to gain weight. He was really "into" looks and became quite disturbed about what was happening to his physique.

One day he came in to see me after being drunk the night before. The first thing that he did was throw up in the bathroom. He came out and said, "I guess it's time to start talking about the alcohol." I sensed that he was at a point where things were ready to fly apart. His wife was concerned about his escalating drinking and that they could not just have a glass of wine. The bottle just seemed to magically disappear. We knew that there were escalating problems.

I knew that in his mind, his model of alcohol and marijuana intake predated what he was actually doing by about two years. We began to spend a lot of time talking about how his alcohol use had increased because of his involvement with cocaine.

Avoiding the Error of Multiple Substance Abuse Models

I lumped the drummer's alcohol and marijuana consumption together. I didn't say, "Let's have one model for alcohol and another model for pot," because this is a tough one to develop a model for. You won't find many people's lives getting out of control on marijuana alone unless they are people who smoke ten joints a day, become totally unmotivated, don't pay the bills, and let their lives fall apart.

We merge the two, the alcohol and the marijuana. We work with the progressive nature of that, setting up parameters for what out of control means. We set up a monitoring system. What I did was ask him, "What does 'out of control' alcohol and marijuana use mean to you?" He gave me these answers: "When I can't practice my drums. When I start to feel physically bad. When I get away from my physical exercise program. When I start to feel badly about myself."

The Odds of Maintaining Control

On an outpatient basis, I can use an approach like the one I used with the drummer. On an inpatient basis, where you are working with abstinence, you can't. The one thing I never tell clients, however, is that it's okay to use alcohol or marijuana. I say the odds are against them if they try, and they will fail. I give them some unpleasant statistics. "During the last five or six years that I have concentrated on cocaine, only a couple of people I've known have been able to go out and resume smoking marijuana and drinking, without going back to cocaine, or ending up with their lives out of control. Only an exceptional few can do it. The odds are stacked against you. You wouldn't bet on a horse at the race track with odds like that. So why bet your life now?"

Group Reactions Reinforce

If the cocaine dependent is involved with other recovering addicts in a therapeutic group, he won't get far with the argument that alcohol and pot are okay. As soon as he starts talking about his ability to smoke marijuana and drink, he will hear from people who just came back to the group from a relapse caused by the same thinking. Then you are going to have the "us and us" taking place—the good modeling from the other patients who have tried it and failed.

Group reactions are powerful in shaping perceptions and changing thought patterns. However, if the client goes out and tries drinking and smoking, and fails, I always avoid saying "I told you so" sorts of things. I make sure that clients always have a direct line back to me. If things start to go wrong for them they have therapeutic permission to call me back to work with them.

The Abstinence Dilemma

This case, while representing the approach I advocate, violates some principles of addiction therapy. I believe that abstinence is the way that works. Yet, if I am too rigid in that belief, I put the person out of a treatment setting. You alienate him from treatment in such a way that things will get much worse before he gets back in and we start to work again. I think that by being flexible here, I minimized the drummer's pain while creating a system that he could intellectually understand.

Let's look at some other problems in applying this model. One problem occurs when you are working in an inpatient unit that insists on abstinence. I reemphasize that in the case of the drummer I worked on an outpatient basis. I couldn't do this in an inpatient setting. Our inpatient units are abstinence based.

How can you frame conditional approval to continue alcohol and pot exploration so that the client won't go back out and say, "My therapist said we're just going to watch my alcohol and marijuana use. You should really change therapists because mine is really hip." How do you deal with this? If they tell you they don't have a problem with alcohol and marijuana, then they shouldn't have a problem *not* using for six months. You contract it. You say, "Let's look at your use over the next thirty days to see if you do have a problem. But for right now you're in this program. The philosophy of this program is abstinence and you are expected not to use."

EUPHORIC RECALL

Next, I would like to describe the internal and external triggers that are involved in rekindling the desire to use cocaine. When you dialogue with the patient, exploring the alcohol and drug issue, start asking the *when, where,* and *what-is-going-on* questions.

I find it helpful to list as many details as I can about when this person uses. "Tell me when you first used. Tell me about the night that you typically used. What night do you start? What is going on then? Are there times when you find yourself more hungry for cocaine than others?" Start to ask innocuous questions; questions that are often the most revealing. "What are you doing for fun? How are things going on in your life? What are you doing over the weekends? How did that go for you when you were using cocaine?"

What you will begin to see is that there is usually a set of internal and external triggers that rekindle cocaine hunger and a return to the drug. Among the important internal events are boredom, stress, and the need for a reward.

One of the things I talk about with clients is *euphoric recall.* With euphoric recall, we remember all the nice things and we put all the nasty things in the misty background. It is a recurring human phenomenon. I look at it this way: Have you ever had someone who severely hurt or damaged you? A friend of yours comes over and says, "Gees, I saw so-and-so the other day." You say, "Yes, I remember him," and then say something nice about him. Then you remember that you hated him. It is the euphoric recall that comes back first.

Cocaine addicts remember the euphoria. The euphoria is firmly implanted. The euphoria starts with anticipating *copping* the drug and "really getting off." This person is high even before they put the drug into their system. It speaks a lot about putting them around the drug.

Triggers to Altered Consciousness

This is an alcohol story but it reveals the importance we place on a chemical. This story is fiction, but mirrors reality. It portrays how we can alter our state of consciousness even with a minuscule amount of a chemical:

> It is a beautiful day in Oak Forest, Illinois, where I live. I am driving home in my paid for car, to my beautiful paid-for house in the suburbs. I pull in the driveway; my two kids run out and give me a big hug and say, "Dad, we're so glad you're home." I'm home for the weekend. It's a beautiful Spring day. I walk into the house and smell a beautiful meal being cooked. I kiss my lovely wife, go to the refrigerator, pull out one can of beer, pop the top, take a swallow, and say, "Boy, do I feel better now."

It wasn't all the marvelous things around me that made me feel better. One swallow of beer did nothing for me physiologically. But it had psychological impact. It altered my state of consciousness in the direction of euphoria. The weekend's started.

Any situation that was strongly attached to the use of cocaine will trigger euphoric recall. Large amounts of money will trigger euphoric recall. "I get paid. It's Friday night and I always get loaded on Friday nights. Now I go to the bank; I have three hundred dollars in my pocket and I'm going home. I'm going through an area near the person I used to buy from. I'm listening to hard rock music on the radio. (The music is an external anchor.) I start to feel strange. The thought comes to my mind that it sure would be nice to have some cocaine now."

Tell the recovering cocaine dependent to expect this to happen. I tell them that there will be times when they will even dream about cocaine. When it happens, look at what is going on in your life. Usually, you'll find that you are going through a high stress time. Look at what you are not doing to maintain your sobriety.

Reverse Rituals

One thing you want to do before clients get out of the treatment center is put them around paraphernalia, so they can deal with an external cue. Have them go through some *reverse rituals*. If they have a freebase pipe, have them go through the ritual of breaking it. Trash the paraphernalia. I have had people tell me that after their first time through treatment, they found themselves scraping the pipe in hopes of finding enough in there to smoke.

I try to get these souvenirs of cocaine addiction out of the way. I think that there is a reason people hang onto them. If they have accepted that they can't use again, it's easy for them to get rid of the pipe. If they "hem and haw" about it, say that they want to keep it to remember past bad times, I worry. There is still a part of them that would like to use cocaine again.

I forecast the times when the client will have difficulty with euphoric recall. We identify events and feeling states that trigger this experience, the high risk situations that they may put themselves in. I try to help the recovering addict anticipate the impact of euphoric recall, and be ready to deal with it without succumbing. Then I initiate mental imagery techniques.

Disassociating

A valuable mental imagery technique is *"disassociating,"* moving someone a little bit away from the experience. Have you ridden a roller coaster? Put yourself mentally back into that situation. You're on the roller coaster going toward the top of the first big hill. You're getting ready to go over the top. Now you're going over the top and you can feel the wind in your hair and you get that rush.

Now change your experience. Put yourself on a bench watching yourself go up to the top of the hill and going down the other side. What is the difference? In the first image you relive the experience. In the second image, you watch yourself do it. If you want a nice associative experience as good as, or better than, a cup of coffee in the morning, associate with the roller coaster ride. Except now make it clearer, faster, and amplify it. You can start to get that adrenalin rush.

One thing you can do when someone is experiencing drug craving is to have him disassociate and watch himself. Ask, "What do you see? What is going on?" Have him start to describe it, because that starts to detach him from the brain processes that are so "tuned into" the experience itself. I find that by having clients practice disassociating it makes it easier for them to handle cravings. Disassociating allows objective viewing of an emotional situation.

If I have people who reach the stage where the craving is so bad that their emotions have completely overridden their intellect, I use an equation. It is: *thoughts + emotion = behavior.* When you have a cocaine addict who is having a lot of difficulty, the one thing he can control is his behavior. We all know how this works. Every time we think and feel something, it influences how we behave at that moment. I think it's interesting to note that if we turn this equation around, if we engage in productive behavior, we alter thoughts and emotions in a positive way.

FINDING ALTERNATIVE REWARDS

I worked with some lawyers who were captivated by reward. They said things like, "When I win a big case I buy cocaine and go to the bar with other lawyers. We do a lot of cocaine and this is my reward. The time I buy is when I win a case." Winning a big case would almost instantly put them into a cocaine hunger. To recover, they had to be aware of that. Then we had to work on alternative responses to winning. Number one—stay out of the bar to begin with. If a big case is coming up, structure a meeting for afterward. Structure a positive activity for that evening, not a self-defeating one.

USING MENTAL IMAGERY EFFECTIVELY

If you do mental imagery with a cocaine addict or a chemically addicted person on an outpatient basis, always do it at the beginning of the session. Mental imagery may trigger some feelings and craving. You want to make sure you can deal with them before that person goes home. Suppose a person has trouble with a particular situation. He or she might say, "Every time I go to a wedding reception, I end up snorting cocaine with my friends and we get crazy all night long." My task is to have that person see himself, in his mind, going into the exact situation in a sober state. Provide alternative behaviors to help deal with euphoric recall. Have clients mentally and behaviorally (verbally) practice the positive alternatives.

There are other things you can do. For example, if recovering cocaine dependents must go into a risky environment make sure they take someone from the program. Make sure they drive themselves—so that they don't go with two other crazies who are going to be snorting cocaine until 4 A.M., leaving them waiting for a ride home. They call this "action planning" or problem solving. Teach them how to create a way out of situations that are dangerous. Give them the power to interrupt the pattern.

NICOTINE, COFFEE, AND DIET PILLS

Another thing that I look at is the other stimulating drugs that cocaine addicts are using. Although accepting cocaine problems, they may be taking diet pills on the side, or have a high intake of caffeine and nicotine. Nicotine is a powerful stimulant. If you snorted nicotine in the same quantities that you snort cocaine it would kill you. It is more toxic. Nicotine is a potent central nervous system stimulant with addictive properties. If there is a tremendous amount of caffeinated coffee and nicotine, they are starting to get that old stimulation, buzz and excitement. I want to curtail that if possible—reduce cigarette smoking and use decaf.

Desensitizing To Cocaine Aroma

Do you know cocaine has a smell?   It is labeled as a white, crystalline, odorless powder.   But when you extract cocaine you often use a solvent (acetone or ether), and it will have a strong and unique odor.   People who freebase and inject will describe the ether vapor smell as distinct for them. They first discovered how profound the smell is about two years ago.

I worked with an anesthesiologist who would only get hungry when he had to go into the operating room. He started to smell the anesthetic and it would "drive him nuts." He didn't understand it until he made the connection that one of his anchors was smell. Ron Siegele, in California, has worked with a synthetic cocaine aroma which can be made by mixing three inert chemicals.   During early recovery, allow the recovering addict to smell that vial *ad lib*. It may have a desensitizing property and it does seem to take away some of the cocaine hunger for some individuals.

WHEN COCAINE IS PART OF A RELATIONSHIP

One issue to consider is whether to work with the "significant other." I always work with the significant other whenever possible. Is cocaine a common denominator in the relationship? This is the first and most important question to ask. If what the couple is giving to one another is cocaine, in a way it is not drastically different from the couple that argues, has a bottle of champagne, goes to bed together, and has a honeymoon for a week. The anxiety builds. They blow up at one another, go out, get drunk and then make love.

Suppose you have a patient who has been in inpatient care and is returning home on a pass. It's the final weekend before discharge and the day is going to be spent with the wife, girlfriend, or whoever. They jump into bed and in five minutes it is all over. They have the euphoric recall of what cocaine did for sex early in the addictive process. You have someone who is recalling that they used to stay up all night long and "get it on."   Now it's over in five minutes. Both of them, or at least one of them, is thinking, "Damn, it would be great to have a gram right now."

It is especially difficult if both parties are cocaine dependent. If this is the case, many new issues arise. They may have emotionally distanced one another. What do you do to enhance their intimacy, to allow them to deal with this issue? Usually there is nothing wrong physiologically. It just has become part of their psychology that every time they have sex they think about cocaine. It's another anchor.

Expanding Dimensions of Sexuality

Can you think of any way to make that intimate relationship just a little bit easier? You can prepare them for this. How can you create a nice romantic evening? There are things that can be done to prolong the evening, to make it rewarding. Carefully planning a romantic evening together helps. This should only be used if there is true caring in the relationship, and only as an adjunct to couples counseling.

I do a little teaching. I explain the fact that people who do a lot of drugs together lose many of the most important parts of sexuality. Sexuality has many layers and tiers. There is caring, inclusion, acceptance, friendship, and genital response. In chemical dependency they lose it from top to bottom. The last thing they lose is the genital response. I start working on the caring, inclusion, acceptance, and friendship. I get them to invest in planning romance, candlelight dinners, nice evenings together. Encourage them to do more foreplay. I find that it helps by prolonging the sexual act. It give them something that is intimate and enjoyable. It also creates excitement in the relationship—which cocaine also did. I find that these simple techniques work better than anything else.

Dealing With Guilt and Shame

One of the issues that you have to deal with is the guilt and shame arising from some of the sexual acts that cocaine addicts engaged in. You will see wife and husband swapping, and group sex. All this is part of the craziness of the cocaine high and cocaine toxicity. If you have a spouse who is also involved, and if you consider the poor judgment associated with cocaine use, you will note cheating and extra-marital affairs. Many recovering cocaine addicts put their marriages "right on the verge" by getting involved in affairs just so they can get the excitement they crave.

Try to treat the family. Get them involved in recovery. Unfortunately, there may be no formal organization in your area that accepts and works with the family problems of the cocaine addict. For example, Al-Anon is an effective family program, but in your area or situation they may not want to deal with the family of a cocaine user. If you do have *Family Anonymous*, it is a reasonably effective alternative. When you work with family recovery you will face all the same issues that are dealt with in any substance abuse or addiction. You may find less denial and more of a "shock" dynamic in the cocaine family.

Chapter 8

PREVENTING RELAPSE

* The Relapse Dynamic
* Changing the Pattern
* Anchors
* Confronting Cocaine Hunger
* High Risk Situations
    -Physical Proximity to Cocaine
    -Familiar Places
    -Boredom and Stress
    -The Hazards of Too Much Cash
    -Managing Cocaine Debt
* Telephone Intervention
* Is Will Power an Option?
* Signs and Symptoms of Resistance
* The Future

Linda had graduated two months ago from a residential treatment program. She had been diagnosed as addicted to both cocaine and alcohol. Her treatment plan included two NA and two AA meetings per week. She also had established a solid nutritional and physical exercise program.

Still, part of Linda yearned for the "high life." One weekend, an old college sorority sister came to town. Linda remembered the sorority, college, the friend—the old party scene. She consented to meet her old friend Marsha at a familiar hangout, "Gary's Duck Inn and Waddle Out." There, Marsha convinced Linda that a few cocktails could never hurt. Besides, her problem really was cocaine, not alcohol. Cocaine was the only thing she had really ever lost control of.

Weeks passed and Linda felt more and more guilty about her lapse. She attended fewer meetings and didn't return her *sponsor's* phone calls. One Friday night—feeling confused and anxious—she again went back to the bar seeking some relief. There she ran into Tom. Tom and Linda had been involved in a cocaine romance prior to her treatment. Although part of her knew better, Tom's offer of coke and sympathy was too much to turn down.

Tom and Linda went back to her place and snorted line after line of cocaine from the mirror. Seduced by the drug and Tom, and unbalanced from not working her recovery program, Linda was *wired* again. She had taken up where she had left off—in the spiral of a blossoming cocaine addiction.

THE RELAPSE DYNAMIC

The relapse dynamic consists of more than just returning to cocaine. We know an alcoholic's relapse often begins with a marijuana cigarette. With the cocaine addict, we start to see relapse occur in many ways. I have had patients who would go to Narcotics Anonymous or Alcoholics Anonymous, drink ten cups of coffee, smoke a pack of cigarettes and come out saying, "This is wonderful, I can't wait to get back." They were so "hyped up" they were gathering some of the cocaine experience. When you drink coffee excessively you start to "get off" on it. You get a little shaky and talkative. Your adrenalin level rises and you smoke a pack of cigarettes on top of that.

In considering relapse, then, we must look beyond drugs and alcohol. Cocaine dependents reach a point where their world seems to be falling apart. They report feeling like they are going to die, go crazy, or return to drugs. And returning to cocaine is no longer an option. They end up having accidents, physical problems, emotional problems, or even attempt suicide. These phenomena represent a *relapse dynamic.*

CHANGING THE PATTERN

In treating cocaine addicts you repeatedly hear, "When I feel depressed I use. When I am lonely I use. It's Friday night and my intention is not to use cocaine, but I am sitting alone on Friday evening with nothing to do. I feel empty—bored and empty." What thought comes to mind next? "If I use cocaine I won't feel bored and empty."

For example, Martin, a cocaine addict, thought he would never use cocaine again. Not with all that he had learned from his therapist. But, one Saturday night Martin decided that he felt too tired and lonely to go to his home NA meeting. He decided to stay home—to rest and wallow in his isolation. He heard his sponsor's voice saying, "The time to go to a meeting is the time you least feel like going. That's when you need it the most." Martin didn't heed his sponsor's advice.

Around 9:00 P.M. Martin started to play some old music on the stereo, the music he used to play on Saturday night when he stayed at home alone doing cocaine. He noticed that he was feeling anxious and found himself picking up the telephone twice. He was thinking about calling Lance, his former dealer. Each time he resisted the temptation.

As time went by the "blues" kept rolling in. Martin felt as if he had to call Lance, go crazy, or die. All three were non-recovery options. Out of desperation he called Lance, who was all too happy to sell Martin cocaine. You see, Martin and Lance had been lovers and had always done cocaine together. When Martin admitted his problem, Lance had introspected, wondering what this meant in terms of his own cocaine use. Now Lance convinced Martin that neither had a problem. There were many others who had worse habits than they ever had. Those were two problem users.

Structuring time is one way of what is called "changing the pattern." There are recovering cocaine addicts who spend time in their former neighborhoods, meet the same people they used to, and listen to the same music. As part of an effective recovery program, they must change these behaviors. For example, some of us have the "high school Fridays." In high school, Friday night was always my party night. So when I entered college life, Friday was always the hardest night to deal with. If that is the reality of the cocaine person, you must break their pattern of Friday nights. I look for patterns relating to cocaine use and devise ways to change them.

For example, I don't permit a recovering cocaine dependent to leave work on a Friday night with much cash in his pocket. I take away cash station cards and put people on budgets. Money is just another anchor to watch out for. I also say, "What other route can you take home? What different radio station do you have available? I would rather have you take the longer route home, listen to easy listening music, and once you get home, have a structured activity involving self-help, or your family."

ANCHORS

Anchored experience is a concept central to relapse prevention. An example of an anchored experience is chewing aluminum foil on a cavity. Or, have you heard someone take their finger nails and rake them down a chalk board? I don't have to give you the aluminum foil. You have that experience "stashed" in your brain. It's important to remember that the drug experience is similarly "stashed" in the brain of every chemically dependent person.

"When I am hungry, angry, lonely, or tired—I drink or drug." That's what the anchored experience translates to. Of course this idea isn't new. It has been around in the Alcoholics Anonymous literature since the 1930's. I think this is one of the few field's where we can go back into the historical literature and still come up with techniques that are relevant to solving today's problems.

CONFRONTING COCAINE HUNGER

The development of a hunger or craving is characteristic of any drug that is abused. People start to crave it. The craving associated with cocaine dependence is profound. I've often had people call me up and say, "It's the only thing I can think of. I can see a picture in my mind of myself doing cocaine. I can see myself buying it and laying the lines out, filling up the pipe...." They're having an associative experience in which they're actually living it again. When people do that they become very emotional and less intellectual. They are overwhelmed by the profound sense of "I would really like to go out and get some of this drug."

HIGH RISK SITUATIONS

To identify the high risk situations, the most helpful thing you can do is engage in dialogue with a patient. Listen to what they say and they'll tell you when their high risk times are. There will be Friday nights, a lot of Thursday nights, and if they are "really hip" they'll know that their dealer usually "cops" on Wednesday or Thursday night. It's best to get to your dealer then, before the cocaine gets all "cut" up. You get better "stuff." You find out when they "cop," and when they'll be in situations when they'll think about "copping."

Physical Proximity to Cocaine

This is an incredible statistic: eighty-three percent of the recovering cocaine dependents say they just can't resist cocaine if they are near it. "I don't want to use, but if I put myself in physical proximity to cocaine, I can't say 'no' to it." There is a powerful anchor.

Cocaine dependents have a sixth sense. I have found that many can walk into a room and sense everyone in the room who is using. The *Diagnostic and Statistical Manual* of the American Psychiatric Association (DMS-III) missed the boat on that. They talked about adjustment disorders. They have adjustment disorders with depression, anxiety, with mixed features, but they missed one. It is called "adjustment disorder with resentment.

Adjustment disorder with resentment is what happens when you walk into a room where all your friends are using, and you know that you can't. You will be angry, resentful, and emotional—the same things that happen to the alcoholic who picks up three drinks at a wedding reception, notices he's about to drink, and says, "What the hell am I doing?"

Familiar Places

Driving past the dealer's house is an anchor. I learned about this type of anchor from an insurance salesman in Chicago. He told me, "I had to alter my downtown Loop route because every time I went past my old watering hole, I'd start feeling really weird. I'd feel real strange, right in the pit of my stomach." What he found was his own intervention. He stopped going that way. He took a different block, went around the corner, and it alleviated his anxiety. Keep the recovering addict out of places where he doesn't need to be. You can start to break the pattern. By all means he must avoid being around cocaine.

Some people like to test themselves by setting up high risk situations. I hear stories all the time like: "I was just riding in the neighborhood, just happened to be in that area, and I was thinking about my friend Johnny, who I always got my cocaine from. Johnny is a very good friend of mine and I miss having the chance to talk to him.

So I go over to Johnny's house and I notice that as I get one block away from Johnny's house I am gripping the steering wheel so hard my knuckles are white. My car is going a little faster than it usually does. I come screeching into Johnny's driveway and I go inside. In that process I have already convinced myself that it's okay to use cocaine. I can 'blow it off' tomorrow. I can just do it for tonight and worry about it later." Or he may say, "It's okay to snort as long as I stay away from the pipe." Or, "I'll only do a gram and quit by 11 P.M."

The best thing we can do is structure those high risk times with alternative behaviors. You may want to introduce behaviors that are helpful to the family; self-help, fun activities. Work on keeping that person's life balanced. If you can identify the triggers, they usually imply the use of certain types of interventions. Break the pattern; it's fundamental.

Boredom and Stress

Boredom is a big risk. The scenario goes like this: "I worked hard this week and suddenly it's Friday night. I have no social plans. It's 9 P.M. and I'm bored. What I would like is a little excitement." Then I play a little mind game with myself that I've played before. I say, "I'm going to go out and buy a gram. That's all I'm going to use." Then sometime around Sunday, when I have gone through about a quarter of an ounce, I realize that, once again, my scheme didn't work. The solution is to break the old pattern. If boredom sets in on Friday night, structure in an alternative behavior.

What we are defining here are the old patterns. What happens when cocaine addicts are under stress? They use chemicals to maintain internal controls. Although many people use depressant drugs like alcohol when they are under stress, cocaine, a stimulant, may have a calming effect on the addict. The treatment challenge is to help them acquire alternative behavior patterns.

The Hazards of Too Much Cash

Let's consider some external triggers of relapse. A large sum of money is an external trigger. I find that if a cocaine addict gets paid on Friday and he made seven hundred dollars, he will often put two or three hundred dollars in his pocket. So when a client receives a large sum of money, on payday for example, I have him go straight to the bank or, better yet, have the check sent to a bank.

I eliminate bank cards, too, if I can. I go through a ritual of having them broken up and thrown away. I put clients on a budget. By putting them on a budget, they don't have that anchor in the pocket. I try to have them carry no more than thirty or forty dollars in cash. Most people don't need to walk around with more cash than that.

Familiar songs are an external anchor; all the old heroin songs like, "...when you're married to H, you're married for life...." And the British Blues bands—it's like you can just "get down" with them. They alter your state of consciousness. Have you ever heard Eric Clapton's cocaine song? You can "get off" on that song without cocaine. It's an upbeat piece of music and you "get into" that. I try to work with people, especially at high risk times, to tune into easy listening. Listen to a sports station, a talk show. Do something different. Break the pattern.

Managing Cocaine Debt

One precipitator of relapse falls under the category "returning to work." What do you do when you have a client who works for GM and owes two thousand dollars to people who work in the plant? He is just getting ready to leave an inpatient environment and return to the work place. How would you deal with that? What would you do? He's scared and emotional. He knows the people he owes money to are going to come up to him with a deal. "There is a way you can start to pay me back. I have a good deal for you. I got an ounce in my locker and you can cut a couple grams out for yourself, if you like, and sell the rest."

How do you deal with that? You help cocaine dependents develop alternative responses to this problem through role playing. One alternative response is to make arrangements to pay off the debt. I think that taking the initiative is the best tool here. They usually have the phone numbers of the people they owe money. While they're still in treatment I have them telephone the people they owe money to and make arrange-ments to repay the debt. "I will pay you so many dollars every paycheck."

There is one thing to be careful of. You don't want them to try to pay back too much, too soon. This causes problems in other areas of life which can trigger relapse—like if they can't pay the rent or feed the kids. You should go through a budg-eting process that will allow them to meet their basic needs, but keep cocaine creditors off their backs.

Despite a strong fear of returning to work, recovering addicts can be shown how to take control of the situation. "I have a plan. Every payday I pay back Joe and Mark twenty-five dollars each." It may take a year or two, but you will see that they do well with this. However, after three or four months they may start resenting having to pay this money back. At least you have "bought them some time," taken the heat off. Then you can start to work with that resentment. The problem evolves, evolves and evolves. Solutions require time.

TELEPHONE INTERVENTION

When someone calls you on the phone and says he's experiencing an irresistible urge to use cocaine, have him try to dissociate. You can do it over the phone. Remember from the last chapter, association is reliving it, or being there. Disassociation is being able to step back and watch yourself and watch what you are doing.

Let me share a story to exemplify this. I want to put a disclaimer on this story. I do not recommend doing this, but in this instance it was all I had to work with.

I had a twenty-seven year old rock musician for a client, who also owned a cattle ranch. I just picked him up from a cardiac care unit. He had freebased thirty-two hundred dollar's worth of cocaine in less than forty-eight hours and they thought he had had a heart attack. It turned out that he was having a cardiac *arrhythmia* with associated chest pain.

He called me up, two days out of the hospital (we had set up an appointment for the next day) and said, "CC, I just can't make it. I think I'm going to kill myself." I said all the injunctions... "It's not okay to kill yourself...," went through all the dialogue, and determined it was *remote ideation*. He had no plan and appeared to be asking for help. So then I said, "M_, I want you to do one thing. I'm on the north side of town and I want you to meet me at my home office. It's thirty minutes away from your house, but it will take me one hour to get there. I want you to clean your living room. (I knew this person was a bachelor and what his house looked like.) Then get in your car and come to see me."

I rushed home, taking forty-five minutes to an hour getting there. I got there, waited for M_, and nothing happened. When I called him he said, "You know what? I cleaned up my living room and I started to feel so good I decided I didn't need to see you."

This story illustrates that through positive behavior we can reshape thoughts and emotions. Any time we are dealing with craving, if we can start to dissociate a little bit and get people into nearly any positive alternative behavior, we can ease the feeling.

IS WILL POWER AN OPTION?

All that will power and self-control do is prolong the agony. Trying to cure cocaine addiction with will power is similar to trying to cure diarrhea with will power. It simply doesn't work. Why doesn't will power work?

I find that patients who have been through treatment two and three times are often working a will power model. They selectively hear only the things that support that model. When they finally begin showing real progress they may be responding to some of the seeds that were planted during earlier treatments. "Oh! I remember!" takes on a new meaning.

In abandoning the will power model, they reach the point where they can say and believe "I'm a cocaine addict." And they can say it three or four times without getting it caught in their throats. People start saying, "Gee, It's not so sad that I'm a cocaine addict because I've had to learn a whole lot. I've had to adjust my lifestyle so that I feel productive. I have something to look forward to in my life."

When I observe clients, I often find the *meta-message*, how they behave, is more important than what they say. Are they comfortable with abstinence? I look at people who work a will power model as having a war going on inside. The most miserable people I have ever seen are addicted people who try to work a will power model. We call it a "dry drunk" or "white knuckle abstinence." There is "a piece in their head" that says "Okay, experience has taught me that I can't do cocaine. But there is still a piece of me that says, 'NO, I AM NOT a cocaine addict.'" There is constant conflict, double messages, and discordance inside the individual.

SIGNS AND SYMPTOMS OF RESISTANCE

I think compliance and resistance stem from the internal turmoil that occurs when a person is working a will power model, instead of "turning it over, to let go and let God." If we look at compliance, which in my mind may be another form of resistance, the body and mind are discordant.

Where is the energy going in this model? The energy is all internal, trying to figure out what is going on. They think, "Every day I feel bad. I feel like I'm on edge all the time. I'm always thinking about using. I got a piece of me that is fueling the hope that maybe I'll be able to use again. I'm not comfortable with me. I am not comfortable in any way."

When I start seeing these things, the words I notice are "I should, I ought, I can, I could." All these are will power words. They imply control over my addiction. "I should be able to control this thing."

Suppose you are starting a treatment plan with someone. You say, "Yes, you should make four meetings a week, and your wife should do this, and we suggest that you go to aftercare for a year." Suppose he starts bargaining with you. This is a sign of resistance. If someone has accepted that he is truly cocaine dependent, he would logically want to use every available modality to deal with this addiction. When a person is unwilling to do that, it is symptomatic of the war inside.

Something positive happens when a person accepts that he is chemically dependent, a cocaine addict. There is congruence between the body and the mind. All his energy can be channeled into a beautiful recovery program. A person can start to move and make things happen in his life. The way he looks is different. The way he talks is different. The words he uses are different. He can say "I'm a cocaine addict," and say it three times and be okay with it.

Finally, my feeling is that people can't relapse until they accept that they have a problem. You're not actually in a recovery program until you've gone through the acceptance stage. You can't relapse from a relapse.

THE FUTURE

Today everyone is concerned about crack and rock cocaine. It may be a purer form of the drug than was available earlier, although this often is not true. From parents, afraid of the impact of this potent drug on the brain, therapists and counselors are constantly hearing the question: "How can I get my son or my daughter off cocaine?"

It's the toughest question in the world, and there's no consoling answer. We don't have a formula to make these kids quit. We don't have a formula to make someone's husband or wife quit. I was once impressed by having a lady stand up during a seminar, as if no one else existed, and say, "My husband left me for cocaine. My life was just ideal a year ago, but today we owe fifty thousand dollars. We have to sell our car, our house...we're in hock up to our ears." She was jilted—and she was jilted by the person she loved for a white inert powder.

When we search for a solution to the cocaine problem we usually turn to demand. I wasn't sure whether to be angry or laugh when I heard the President of Bolivia say that all we need is one hundred million dollars a year for the next four years, and maybe we can put a dent in this problem. You see, *we are not going to stop supply unless we stop demand.*

Urine testing and other maneuvers may be helpful, but while we have families that are dysfunctional, and role models who are chemically dependent or alcoholic—as long as we have people out there who are empty and who see cocaine as a missing piece—we will have a supply of the drug. It's a fast and easy way to make money.

A person can make up to $150,000 just on a contract to use his private plane to fly a shipment of cocaine under radar. When you look at those sums of money, you see bankers and business people becoming involved. There was a big bust in Philadelphia—all lawyers and doctors and dentists—who had been the principal suppliers of cocaine to the area since 1978. When you look at a bust of forty-six hundred pounds, and realize that cocaine is at least five times as valuable as gold, you begin to appreciate the magnitude of the cocaine economy.

What does this imply for crime? You're an adolescent who wants to break out of a low socio-economic area. You notice the person in your neighborhood who has the good clothes and expensive car—your role model, sometimes—and you look at the baseball players, and basketball and football players. When they are involved with cocaine, what will you conclude about how to succeed in life?

We've had ball players come out of treatment programs, and the next week they're on TV saying, "Kids, don't use drugs." And then, the following week, they are back in treatment, and then they are out playing. And this happens two or three times. They relapse, they play; they relapse, they play—and they make a million dollars a year. Now what do you conclude from that? The way to get what you want, the way to get out of this environment—the way to wealth and fame—the way to have the types of friends you want, and the way to material possessions is through the drug economy.

I'm thankful that someone told me that the value of the baseball cards, of the players who were in the Peter Uberoth investigation for cocaine, has gone down in the eyes of our children. There is some hope. I think that Ronald and Nancy Reagan making statements like 'drugs are public enemy number one' is a positive act. We have some good role models coming out and saying, "Hey, there is a better way of life"—what self-help is calling the "easier, softer way of life"—a program where there is an intersection between our relationship with God and our relationship with our fellow man. That's the point in The Cross called spirituality.

Appendix A

"Controlled Substances Act"
Comprehensive Drug Abuse Prevention and Control Act of 1970
P.L. 91-513

An Overview of Legal Aspects

In 1970 the United States federal government enacted the Controlled Substances Act which established five categories or "schedules" listing potentially abused medications.

SCHEDULE I:
Highest potential for abuse with no recognized medical use except for experimental purposes.

    Example - Heroin, LSD, Marijuana, and Pep

    Penalties - First offense penalties for trafficking in Schedule I drugs range from 5-15 years with a $15,000-$25,000 fine

SCHEDULE II:
High potential for abuse but have legitimate medical uses.

    Example - Barbiturates, Amphetamines, Cocaine, and narcotics (Morphine, Demerol, etc.)

    Penalties - Same as Schedule I

SCHEDULE III:
Moderate potential for abuse (low to moderate potential for physical dependence or high potential for psychological dependence); with legitimate medical uses.

    Example - Nonamphetamine type stimulants and nonbarbiturate sedatives (Quaaludes are Schedule II)

    Penalties - Trafficking involves a 5-year sentence and a $15,000 fine for first offense

SCHEDULE IV:
Low abuse potential with limited likelihood of creating physical or psychological dependence.

>   Example - Darvon; some sedatives and pain killers that do not contain narcotics

>   Penalties - Trafficking involves 3-year sentence and $10,000 fine

SCHEDULE V:
Low potential for abuse and may lead to limited physical or psychological dependence.

>   Example - Drugs containing small amounts of narcotics and are used for cough and diarrhea

>   Penalties - Trafficking penalties are one year and a $5,000 fine

GLOSSARY

Acceptance: Often called surrender in self-help groups, this term is the opposite of will power. Acceptance means willingness to admit that our life is out of control, and that we need the help of a higher power (some power outside of ourselves) to lead us from the insanity of drug or alcohol addiction. See Will Power.

Addiction: Loss of control of the intake of alcohol or drugs with continued use despite adverse consequences.

Addictionologist: Medical term for a specialist in the treatment of addictionology.

Adult Children: Those who encountered developmental difficulties growing up in an alcoholic or chemically dependent family.

Adulterant: See Cut

Alcoholics Anonymous (AA): A fellowship of men and women who share their hopes, strengths and experiences with each other such that they help each other in recovery. AA is a support group for primarily alcoholics and is not to be confused with professional treatment.

Amphetamine: A central nervous system stimulant with sympathomimetic effects; common ingredient in prescription diet pills used in the 60's and 70's. Cocaine is pharmacologically very similar to amphetamines.

Amphetamine Psychosis: A condition sometimes occuring among amphetamine users, typically after high dose. Consists of delirium, hallucinations and persecutory delusions.

Anchored Experience: A past experience that can be triggered by being in a similar set or setting. See Internal and External Cues.

Anchors: See Internal and External Cues

Anhedonia: Inability to feel pleasure; a common symptom of Parkinson's disease.

Arrhythmia: An irregular rhythm, often describing heart problem (i.e., cardiac arrhythmia).

Aversive Conditioning: A psychological term for associating a former pleasurable experience, like using cocaine, with a negative consequence.

Benzodiazepines: A pharmacological class of tranquilizing drugs; examples include Valium, Librium, and Xanax.

Blow: A street name for cocaine.

Bust: To be "busted" or caught for possession or distribution of an illegal substance.

Carbacaine: An anesthetic used in medicine that has a "freeze" similar to cocaine. It can be used as an adulterant or "cut."

Cocaine: A central nervous system stimulant with profound sympathomimetic effects; it can be insufflated (snorted), given intravenously (injected), or inhaled through the lungs (free based). See Cocaine HC1, Freebase, I.N. and I.V.

Cocaine Anonymous (CA): A new fellowship, comprised of persons addicted to cocaine, that follows the 12-step program of Alcoholics Anonymous.

Cocaine Bugs: A true halluciation first described in 1889 in Paris, France by Dr. Magnan. Also called Magnan's sign, formication, or parasitosis. Usually seen in high dose chronic uses, the user believes there are bugs under the skin. See True Hallucination.

Cocaine HC1: When the alkaloid cocaine is mixed with an acid (HC1) the product yielded is cocaine HC1, the highly water soluble compound used for insufflation (snorting) or intravenous (I.V.) administration.

Cocaine Psychosis: Typically reversible psychiatric condition characterized by loss of reality. In extreme cases it can mimic paranoid shizophrenia. See Paranoid Schizophrenic.

Contingency Contracting: A contract with a recovering addict where a negative or positive consequence is attached to the addict's fulfillment of agreed upon stipulations.

Copping: Procuring a drug for consumption, in this case cocaine.

Coming Down: When the blood levels of cocaine are decreasing and the user starts to experience what is often described as "anguish."

Crack: Term describing the sound that cocaine makes when it is smoked or freebased.

Crank: A term that often means a state of stimulation of the brain, as in "cranked up" or "wired."

Cravings: Also called drug hunger, a desire to use a drug such as cocaine often in order to alleviate subjective distress.

Cut: Substance added to cocaine to increase volume and weight and to increase profitability. The two typical types of cut include: 1) Inert sugars - Example: inositol, added to increase volume and weight; 2) Other anesthetics - Example: lidocaine, added to give the characteristic anesthetic 'freeze,' in addition to increasing volume and weight.

Cyclothymic Disorder: A disorder of affect or mood involving periods of depression or hypomania.

D.T.s: Delirium Tremens

Denial: A psychological defense system used to help an individual disavow reality.

Dependence: Used interchangeably with addiction. See Addiction.

Disassociating: Acting as if one were a spectator to one's own subjective experience, allowing one to be more objective about an emotional experience.

Dopamine: A neurotransmitter or brain chemical involved in both the pleasurable experience of the cocaine high and the dysphoria of "coming off" of it.

Drug-a-logues: The telling of drug related stories. This typically happens in early recovery when addicts have very little recovery history to discuss.

Dual Diagnosis: Category describing an individual with two disorders. In the context of this book it refers to a diagnosis of chemical dependency along with an existing psychiatric diagnosis (Example: depression).

Dysphoria: Feeling bad.

Dysphoric Rebound: After a euphoric mood a person may have an alternating effect of dysphoria as the blood level of cocaine diminishes.

Edge: Refers to side effects such as tight muscles and grinding teeth, which detract from the euphoric experience.

Eight-ball: Street term for an eighth of an ounce of cocaine.

Electroencephalogram: A measurement of brain wave activity.

Euphoric Recall: The kinesthetic (emotional) recall of the positive aspects of drug use. May be accompanied by physiological signs such as increased heart rate and perspiration.

External Cues: A part of the total drug experience (see Total Drug Experience), incorporating the setting or environmental influences upon the individual. AA often refers to the External People, Places and Things.

Freebase: A smokeable form of cocaine.

Freebasing: The act of smoking cocaine whereby vapors are inahled directly into the lungs. At 6-8 seconds, this is the most rapid way of getting cocaine into the system.

Freeze: An anesthetic or numbing effect.

Haldol: An antipsychotic medication.

Hallucinations: Seeing, hearing or feeling things that in fact do not exist.

Head Magazine: Magazine that contains advertisements for drug related paraphernalia, typically for mail order.

Hit: A unit dose of cocaine. Can be a "line" of cocaine for snorting, a syringeful of cocaine for injecting, or a "rock" of cocaine for freebasing.

Hotshot: An injection of a drug other than the drug expected, or an injection where the purity is greater than that expected.

Hyperkinesia: A disorder with inappropriate degrees of attention, impulsiveness and hyperactivity; an attention deficit disorder.

Hyperpyrexia: Elevated, above normal body temperature. In the cocaine addict's body temperatures may escalate as high as 107 to 108 degrees. If not properly controlled, over time this can be lethal.

Hypersomnia: A lethargic, sleepy state often found in early abstinence from cocaine.

I.N.: See Intranasal

Intranasal (I.N.): The intranasal use of cocaine, by insufflation or "snorting" of cocaine into the nose for absorption by the nasal membranes.

Inositol: A popular inert "cut" added to increase weight and volume—and profits.

Inpatient: A treatment setting where patients live 24-hours a day in a hospital or residential unit.

Inpatient Rehabilitation: Professionally regulated treatment usually lasting three to four weeks. May be hospital or residential-based.

Insufflation: The inhaling through the nostrils of cocaine; also called "snorting."

Intensive Outpatient Program: A program designed to clinically supply the treatment modalities found in a more restrictive inpatient environment, minus the supportive milieu.

Internal Cues: A part of the total drug experience; cues incorporating the "set" or psychological make-up of the individual, psychological make-up being influenced by past experience and expectation. See Total Drug Experience.

Intravenous (I.V.): Intravenously using cociane, i.e., injecting cocaine in solution into the venous system.

I.V.: See Intravenous

Kindling: A type of reverse tolerance to cocaine. Overdose phenomena——like seizures——are experienced at a lower dose than typically tolerated.

Kinky: Unusual or bizarre (as in the sexual practice of bondage under the influence of cocaine).

Lidocaine: A popular cocaine "cut" that has the characteristic numbing and freezing sensation of cocaine. See Cut.

Lithium: A prescribed medication often used to treat bi-polar illness, or manic depression.

Manic-depressive: A psychiatric condition characterized by depressive and manic mood sweeps, more correctly called bi-polar disorder.

Matures Out: A tendency to quit a certain activity with age. Many heroin addicts "mature out" of their use of heroin in their mid-to-late thirties.

Meta-message: The true message.

Monito: A baby laxative that looks just like cocaine and is often used as a "cut" or adulterant. See Cut.

Motivational Crisis: A crisis that escalates pain levels in the cocaine addict such that treatment may be considered an alternative or an imperative. This crisis is often financial or legal.

Nanogram: A very small unit of measure; 1/1000 of a gram.

Nanogram Percent: The number of nanograms of a substance found in 100 ml of blood.

Narcissism: In this context we are referring to "specialness" or "uniqueness" that is part of the cocaine addict's self-perception in early treatment.

Narcissistic Personality Disorder: When narcissistic tendencies are exaggerated and cause problems with the individual's ability to function. Refer to the *Diagnostic and Statistical Manual III* of the American Psychiatric Association.

Narcotics Anonymous (NA): A self-help organization that provides support for recovering drug addicts.

Narcs: Undercover police officers

Neurotransmitters: Chemicals found in the brain and body that are responsible for the continuing transmission of nerve impulses.

Norepinephrine: A stimulatory neurotransmitter, also called Noradrenaline. See Neurotransmitters.

Nuking (the cocaine): The use of a microwave oven as a heat catalyst for the conversion of cocaine HC1 into freebase.

Ounce: A unit dose of cocaine, made up of 28 grams.

Outpatient Treatment: Typically involves the patient living at home while attending treatment services. Outpatient services have varying degrees of service intensity. See Intensive Outpatient Program.

Outpatient Therapy: Professional therapy provided on a least restrictive basis such that client or patient lives at home and utilizes a treatment center one or more times per week.

Parallel Treatment: A treatment strategy used when two disorders occur within one individual, which incorporates the belief that both disorders must be treated somewhat simultaneously, instead of one at a time. See Dual Diagnosis.

Paranoia: A psychological state that may involve a person perceiving that others are out to harm them.

Paranoid Schizophrenic: A psychiatric condition characterized by paranoia in conjunction with a thought and emotional disorder; can lead to violent action.

PCP: Phencylidine, a mood altering illegal drug; sometimes mixed with freebase (space base).

pH: The degree of alkalinity or acidity of the body fluids.

Placebo Effect: Experience of a drug's effect (pain-killing, euphoria-producing, etc.) in a situation where the person believes he is taking a powerful drug but, in reality, is not.

Polydrug: Meaning more than one drug; term typically used to describe a user of more than one type of psychoactive substance, either concurrently or sequentially.

Procaine: An anesthetic sometimes used to "cut" or adulterate cocaine. See Cut.

Professional Treatment: Describes a professionally regulated therapy, such as inpatient rehabilitation or outpatient therapy.

Pseudo Hallucination: When an individual perceives sensations (auditory, visual, or kinesthetic) which they know, intellectually, do not exist. See Snow Lights.

Quaaludes: A hypnotic or sleep-producing drug. Although removed from the U.S. market, may still be obtained illegally.

Reefer: Marijuana

Relapse: A return to the use of alcohol and/or drugs; also refers to a process in early recovery where a patient builds up to the use of alcohol or a drug.

Remote Ideation: A vague idea, as opposed to an immediate well-defined plan.

Reverse Rituals: Reversing the old drug-related rituals (i.e., instead of using the pipe to smoke cocaine, taking the pipe and ceremoniously destroying it).

Rock: Term describing the appearance of cocaine that is smoked or freebased.

Running Set: Persons of similar drug-using habits making up the addict's social support system.

Rush: The experience of "getting off" on a drug; a time when there is an escalating blood level of a drug, experienced by the user as pleasurable.

Score: To "cop" or procure a drug.

Seizure: An electrical overreaction of the brain that can be caused by toxic doses of the powerful brain stimulant cocaine.

Self-Help: Describes any of the supportive type of fellowships such as Alcoholics Anonymous (AA), Narcotics Anonymous (NA), or Cocaine Anonymous (CA).

Serotonin: A neurotransmitter that is involved in sleep and mood control; it is depleted by chronic cocaine use.

Set, Setting: See Internal Cues

Shake and Bake: A street method for converting cocaine HC1 into freebase.

Shoot: To inject a drug directly into a vein.

Slab: Term used for crack and rock or freebase. Instead of being a one-unit dose, the slab is a multiple dose amount in one chunk.

Snorting: See Insufflation

Snow: Another colloquial or "street" term for cocaine.

Snow Lights: A pseudo hallucination often described by chronic cocaine addicts as silver or white specks or geometric forms, typically seen in the peripheral visual field. See Pseudo Hallucination.

Space Base: The combination of PCP with freebase. See PCP and Freebase.

Speedball: The combination of cocaine with heroin; typically injected but may be combined and smoked.

Sponsor: Former addict who is capable of helping a newly recovering addict via support, advice, and modeling.

Stash: An amount of cocaine intended for the personal use of the consumer, and not meant for resale (often referred to as a "personal stash").

Status Epilepticus: A medical condition where there is not one isolated seizure, but life threatening repeated seizures.

Strobing: A condition caused by high dose cocaine administration where there is a flickering of the visual images perceived by the eye.

Sublimation: Substitution

Sympathomimetic: Cocaine's ability to mimic the effects of the sympathetic nervous system on the body, or the "fight or flight" nervous system. See Amphetamine and Cocaine.

Thorazine: An anti-psychotic prescription medication.

Titrate: The mixing of combinations of mood altering substances to establish a desired effect.

Toot: Another term for cocaine, often used in reference to snorting or insufflation of cocaine.

Torch: To light or to heat with a match or other source of fire.

Total Drug Experience (TDE): An individual's subjective experience when they consume a mind altering substance. TDE incorporates the direct pharmacologic effect with the internal and external cues. See Internal and External Cues.

Tricyclic Anti-Depressant: A prescription medication used to treat depression.

Tryptophan: An essential or necessary amino acid often used in treatment of cocaine addiction to restore depleted Serotonin.

True Hallucination: When the individual perceives sensations (auditory, visual, kinesthetic) that are intellectually believed to be real.

Tyrosine: An amino acid which may be used to expedite the replacement of neurochemical deficits during early recovery.

Unit Dose: One dose.

Vena Cava: The large vein entering the right side of the heart.

Will Power: The belief that, "If I were strong enough and tough enough, I '...should...could...can...' deal with this drug or alcohol problem by myself." Opposite of surrender or acceptance. See Acceptance.

Wired: Suffering from the grating side effects of stimulant drugs like cocaine and amphetamines.

BIBLIOGRAPHY

Adler, Patricia A. *Wheeling and Dealing: An Ethnography of an Upper-Level Drug Dealing and Smuggling Community.* New York: Columbia University Press, 1985.

Ashley, Richard. *Cocaine: Its History, Uses and Effects.* New York: Warner Books, 1976.

American Psychiatric Association. *Diagnostic and Statistical Manual III (DSM III).* Washington, D.C.: American Psychiatric Association, 1980.

Anglin, Lise. *Cocaine: A Selection of Annotated Papers from 1880 to 1984 Concerning Health Effects.* Toronto: Addiction Research Foundation, 1985.

Baum, Joanne. *One Step Over The Line: A No-Nonsense Guide to Reorganizing and Treating Cocaine Dependency.* San Francisco: Harper & Row, 1985.

Beckhard, Arthur J., and William D. Crane. *Cancer, Cocaine and Courage; The Story of Dr. William Halsted.* New York: Julio Messner, Inc., 1900.

Brecher, E. *Licit and Illicit Drugs: The Consumers Union Report on Narcotics, Stimulants, Inhalants, Hallucinogens and Marijuana, Including Caffeine, Nicotine and Alcohol.* New York: Little, Brown, 1972.

Brink, Carla J., ed. *Cocaine: A Symposium.* Madison: Wisconsin Institute on Drug Abuse, 1985.

Britt, D. *The All-American Cocaine Story.* Minneapolis, MN: CompCare Publications, 1984.

Cocaine Papers: From Freud to Freebase. rev. ed. Phoenix, AZ: Do It Now Foundation, 1986.

Cocaine Use in America: Epidemiological and Clinical Perspectives. Brooklyn, NY: Revisionist Press, 1986.

Cohen, Sidney. *Cocaine: The Bottom Line.* Washington, D.C.: American Council on Drug Education, 1985.

The Coke Book: The Complete Reference to the Users and Abuses of Cocaine. New York: Berkley Pub., 1984.

Einstein, S. *The Use and Misuse of Drugs.* Belmont, CA: Wadsworth Publishing, 1970.

Eiswirth, Nancy A., Davie E. Smith and Donald R. Wesson. "Cocaine: Champagne of Uppers." *Uppers and Downers.* Englewood Cliffs, NJ: Prentice-Hall, 1973.

Ellinwood, Everett H. "Amphetamines and stimulus drugs." In *Drug Use in America; Problem in Perspective.* Vol. 1, National Commission on Marijuana and Drug Abuse. Washington, D.C.: GPO, 1973.

Emboden, William A., Jr. *Narcotic Plants.* New York: Macmillan, 1972.

Englemann, Jeanne M. *Cocaine: Beyond the Looking Glass Discussion Guide.* Center City: Hazelden, 1984.

Erickson, Patricia, G. *The Steel Drug: Cocaine in Perspective.* Lexington, MA: Lexington Books, 1987.

Gold, Mark S. *Eight Hundred-COCAINE.* New York: Bantam Books, 1984.

Grinspoon, Lester, and James B. Bakalar. *Cocaine: A Drug and Its Social Evolution.* rev. ed. New York: Basic Books, 1985.

Hafen, Brent Q. and Kathryn J. Frandsen. *Cocaine.* Center City, MN: Hazelden, 1982.

Hyde, Margaret O. *Addictions.* New York: McGraw-Hill, 1978.

Johanson, Chris-Ellyn. *Cocaine: A New Epidemic.* Edgemont, PA: Chelsea House, 1986.

Jones, E. *The Life and Work of Sigmund Freud.* New York: Basic Books, 1961.

Kahn, E. J. *The Big Drink: The Story of Coca-Cola.* New York: Random House, 1960.

Kennedy, Joseph. *Coca Exotica: The Illustrated Story of Cocaine.* New York: Cornwall Books, 1985.

Keys, T. E. *The History of Surgical Anesthesia*. New York: Dover, 1963.

Learn About Cocaine. Center City, MN: Hazelden, 1983.

Lee, David. *Cocaine Handbook*. Berkeley, CA: And-Or Press, 1981.

Long, Robert Emmet, ed. *Drugs and American Society*. New York: Wilson, 1985.

Mariani, Angelo. *Coca and Its Therapeutic Application*. 2d ed. New York: J. N. Jaros, 1892.

Meyers, Annie C. *Eight Years in Cocaine Hell*. Chicago: St. Luke Society Press, 1902.

Mills, James. *The Underground Empire: Where Crime and Governments Embrace*. Garden City, NY: Doubleday, 1986.

Mortimer, W. G. *Peru History of Coca, The Divine Plant of The Incas, With an Introductory Account of the Incas and of the Andean Indians of Today*. New York: J. H. Vail & Co., 1901.

Moser, Brian. *The Cocaine Eaters*. New York: Taplinger, 1967.

Musto, David F. *The American Disease: Origins of Narcotic Control*. New Haven and London: Yale Univ. Press, 1973.

National Clearinghouse for Drug Abuse Information. *Cocaine*. Report Series 11, No. 1. Washington, D.C.: GPO, 1971.

O'Connell, Kathleen R. *End of the Line: Quitting Cocaine*. Philadelphia: Westminster, 1985.

Peterson, Robert C., and Richard Stillman, eds. *Cocaine, 1977*. Washington, D.C.: Dept. of Health, Education and Welfare, 1977.

Phillips, Joel, and R. D. Wynne. *Cocaine: The Mystique and the Reality*. New York: Avon Books, 1980.

Plasket, Bruce J., and Ed Quillen. *The White Stuff*. New York: Dell, 1985.

Ray, D. S. *Drugs, Society and Behavior*. St. Louis: C.V. Mosby, 1972.

Rozel, Nicholas J., and E. H. Adams. *Cocaine Use in America: Epidemiological and Clinical Perspectives*. National Institute on Drug Abuse Monograph No. 61. Washington, D.C.: GPO, 1985.

Sabbag, Robert. *Snowblind: A Brief Career in the Cocaine Trade*. New York: Bobbs Merrill, 1976.

Smart, Richard. *The Snow Papers: A Memoir of Illusion, Power-Lust and Cocaine*. Edited by J. Johnson. Boston: Atlantic Monthly, 1985.

Sparkman, J.C., Jr. *The Cocaine Handbook*. Jacksonville Beach, FL: Creative Alternatives Press, 1985.

Spotts, James V., and Franklin C. Shontz. *Cocaine Users: A Representative Case Approach*. New York: Free Press, 1980.

Stone, Nannette, Marlene Fromme, and Daniel Kogan. *Cocaine: Seduction and Solution*. New York: C. N. Potter, 1984.

Sutphen, Trenna. *Final Cut: A Life Changing Self-Help Program to Quit Cocaine*. Malibu, CA: Trenna Productions, 1984.

Tiebout, Harry M., M.D. "Surrender versus Compliance in Therapy." *Quarterly Journal of Studies on Alcohol* 14 (1953): 58-68.

Treating the Cocaine Abuser. Center City: Hazelden, 1985.

Webster, Terry. *Needing Cocaine*. Center City: Hazelden, 1985.

Weil, Andrew. *Chocolate to Morphine*. Boston: Houghton Mifflin, 1983.

———. *The Natural Mind*. Boston: Houghton Mifflin, 1972.

Weiner, Michael A. *Getting Off Cocaine; 30 Days to Freedom: The Step-By-Step Program of Nutrition and Exercise*. New York: Avon, 1984.

Wisotsky, Stephen. *Breaking the Impasse in the War on Drugs*. New York: Greenwood Press, 1986.

Woodley, Richard. *Dealer: Portrait of A Cocaine Merchant*. New York: Holt, Rinehart & Winston, 1971.

Wynn Associates. *Cocaine: Summaries of Psychosocial Research*. Rockville, MD: National Institute on Drug Abuse, 1977.

INDEX